Safe in the Sun

Safe in the Sun

Mary-Ellen Siegel, M.S.W.

Foreword by Albert M. Lefkovits, MD

Walker and Company New York, NY

First published in the United States of America in 1990 by Walker Publishing Company, Inc.

Published simultaneously in Canada by Thomas Allen & Son Canada, Limited, Markham, Ontario

Library of Congress Cataloging-in-Publication Data

Siegel, Mary-Ellen.
    Safe in the sun / Mary-Ellen Siegel : foreword by Albert M.
Lefkovits.
    Includes bibliographical references.
    ISBN 0-8027-1100-6.—ISBN 0-8027-7338-9 (pbk.)
    1. Skin—Care and hygiene. 2. Skin—Cancer—Popular works.
3. Eye—Diseases and defects—Popular works. 4. Solar radiation—
Health aspects—Popular works. I. Title.
RL87.S55   1990
616.5—dc20   90-11947
                                                                    CIP

Printed in the United States of America

2 4 6 8 10 9 7 5 3

To those who provide the sunshine in my life:
my husband Walter
and each of our children
and
grandchildren
Ephram, Eli, Matthew, David, Jonathan, Joshua,
Tzippy, and Samantha

Contents

Chapter 14

A Note to the Reader

Foreword

Until relatively recent times, people of fashion protected their skin from the sun. Only those who had to work outdoors, such as field workers, exhibited signs of chronic sun exposure. In the early 1920s, the famous designer Coco Chanel, returning from a vacation in the sun created a new fashion, making the suntan a desirable end in itself. The bronzed, tanned look soon became identified with the leisure class who could afford to follow the sun year round.

After World War II, travel became accessible to the less affluent who then sought to vacation in the Mediterranean, Caribbean and other places where a suntan was assured. Dermatologists became alarmed as impressive evidence accumulated over the past thirty years linking sun exposure to premature aging of the skin and to the increase in skin cancer throughout the world.

In this comprehensive book, Mary-Ellen Siegel presents information culled from the findings of leading dermatologists and ophthalmologists that demonstrate the link between sun exposure and damage to the skin and eyes. In addition, she explains how people can enjoy the outdoors but still protect themselves, and what can be done to repair any damage that has already occurred. This information is presented in a clear fashion, making it of great value to the general public. I commend this as a means of helping people cope with our changing environment.

Albert M. Lefkovits, M.D.
Assistant Clinical Professor of Dermatology
Mount Sinai School of Medicine, New York
Member, Skin Cancer Foundation Medical Council

Acknowledgments

A number of people are always available to give of their time and expertise when I am writing a book. Some read portions of the manuscript; others tell me of their experiences; still others just stand by and listen while I try to work out details; and countless others, by word and deed, give their support. I am most grateful to all of them.

They include members of the faculty of the Division of Social Work, Department of Community Medicine; the staff of the Levy Library at the Mount Sinai School of Medicine; the staff of the Hillcrest Branch of the Queensborough Public Library, and Dr. Steven Rozenberg of 10/10 Optics.

Ezra M. Greenspan, MD, Lyn Ratner, MD, Bernard Simon, MD, and Michael Wartels, MD, answered questions and made helpful suggestions.

Beth Walker's patience, enthusiasm, and suggestions are enormously appreciated. Steven Gray's contributions were extremely helpful, as were Helen Driller's.

Mitzi Moulds and her staff of the Skin Cancer Foundation were enormously helpful. Joyce Weisbach-Ayoub, Public Information Director, was far more than an important resource: she was always right there when I needed her, providing encouragement and suggestions as well as information.

My family, as always, encourages and sustains me. All of them are very important to me, but in the preparation of this book I owe a special debt of gratitude to my husband's daughter, Jacqueline S. Lustgarten, MD, associate clinical professor of ophthamology at the Mount Sinai School of Medicine in New York. Drafted—rather than politely asked—to look over the sections on eyes, she took on the assignment with characteristic good nature and the same high level of care she extends to her patients, making suggestions and changes.

Albert M. Lefkovits, MD, assistant clinical professor of dermatology at the Mount Sinai School of Medicine in New York, gave of his time and expertise, for which I am most appreciative.

People often wonder how we choose our careers. As a psychotherapist, medical social worker, and health writer, I was inspired by my father, Monroe E. Greenberger, MD, a caring urologist and excellent communicator, and by my mother, a natural and trained healthcare giver who also had the ability to tell a good story. Sharing health information with the public has also become a way of returning the gifts I was fortunate enough to receive from some physicians in my childhood and adolescence. Pediatrician Milton I. Levine, MD, provided wonderful care for me, and later for my children. Three physicians, no longer here, are often in my thoughts: dermatologist Charles Rein, MD; pulmonary specialist George Ornstein, MD; and cardiothoracic surgeon Robert E. Gross, MD. Without them, I would have had no chance to write this or other books. They, along with my father and Dr. Levine, have indelibly shaped my ideas of the values and practices to which healthcare professionals should subscribe.

Introduction

My father began taking home movies long before it was fashionable, and my sister and I have since transferred these to video tape. Now it is possible, in just a few short hours, to watch ourselves grow from infancy to maturity. Viewing these movies one afternoon confirmed what we had long suspected: our lives were one summer, birthday, and sleigh-riding event after another. Birthdays were indoors, but summers found us basking on the beach or ducking the waves on Long Island, and winters appeared to be spent on the snow-covered hills of New York's Central Park. Our sun-kissed faces were a clear indication—so it seemed in those days—of robust health and the advantages of the good life.

Now we know better. Those days of sun-worshiping have put us at risk for skin cancers and melanoma. Today we have the good sense to stop seeking a tan, but until very recently we continued to sit or lie unprotected in the sun. Even after dermatologists began warning against the harm of overexposure to the sun, we (like many of our friends) tended to ignore it. How could anything that made us look so attractive and feel so good be bad for us?

The evidence is in. The sun at the least causes premature aging and wrinkles, and at the worst may contribute to the development of melanoma, a form of skin cancer that can spread throughout the body. Back in the 1930s, the risk of developing malignant melanoma was 1 in 1,500. Now the lifetime risk is 1 in 128. According to the Skin Cancer Foundation, at the current rates of increase, the risk will become 1 in 90 by the year 2000. Although methods of early detection and prompt treatment are available, late stages of malignant melanoma are extremely dangerous. Of the 27,000 known cases of malignant melanoma developed in the United States in 1989. In the same year 6,000 people died of the disease.

Nonmelanoma skin cancer is the most commonly occurring cancer in Caucasian-Americans; over 500,000 new cases are diagnosed each year. About 80 percent of these skin cancers are basal cell carcinomas, and the remaining 20 percent are squamous cell carcinomas. Most of these cancers are curable—especially if treated promptly—but more than 2,000 people died from them last year.

Skin cancer *can* be prevented, and although the effects of the sun are cumulative, you can still reduce the risks by starting to take proper precautions now. Careful and frequent self- and dermatologist-screening greatly increases the likelihood of detection and treatment, with the higher probability of a complete cure.

In the spring of 1988, the American Academy of Dermatology and the Avon Foundation sponsored a national survey of fashion leaders. It revealed that the deep tan once thought to be so glamorous no longer enjoys such esteem. Models are cautioned not to get a suntan anymore, and coworkers no longer think that you must have sat cooped up in your apartment for two weeks if you return from a vacation without a tan.

You can still delight in summer and winter sports. There are ways to be safe in the sun without giving up the many pleasures to be derived from it. The following chapters describe the benefits of sunshine, the risks of exposure, and how damage that has already occurred can be treated or reversed. But most important, we will discuss how you can protect yourself from the sun's damage.

Mary-Ellen Siegel, M.S.W.
January 1990

I

Effects of the Sun

1

What's All the Fuss About?

My grandmother always wore a hat or carried a parasol when she ventured out for long in the sun. She was very proud of her lovely pale skin, which made it clear that she didn't spend her days working in the fields. My mother was born just after the turn of the century. When she married my father in 1924, it was just becoming fashionable to have a suntan—proof that she didn't have to sit over a sewing machine in a factory, and even had the leisure to enjoy a honeymoon in the sun.

I grew up in the 1940s, when it was stylish to return to school in September with a few extra freckles or a suntan, as evidence of parents' ability to provide a fun-filled outdoor summer. During the 1960s and 1970s, when my children were at school, students returning from Christmas or Spring Break with a tan were perceived as being privileged enough to have spent their vacation basking in the Caribbean or skiing at Aspen. One not-so-affluent parent even reported that her teenager asked her to buy a sunlamp so that she could pretend she had been away.

It wasn't unusual for a teenager to choose an outdoor summer job because it offered an opportunity to "work on a tan," and I well remember the love affair we all had with convertibles as still another chance to enjoy the sun.

A tan looked good, and so Caucasians of all ages found ways to get one. And because it looked good, people were convinced that it was good for them, too. We thought the way to dry up a spring or summer cold was to go out in the sun. And when my children were small, I and the mothers with whom I sat in the park always sought out a sunny bench, assuring ourselves that we were giving our babies an extra natural dose of vitamin D.

So what's all the fuss about? "Sure," you may think, "the sun can give me skin cancer, and it can age my skin, but not for a while; and besides, skin cancer is curable. With all those new methods of turning back the clock, it will be a long time before I *look* old."

Not so, the experts tell us. People are incurring skin cancer at younger and younger ages. Even teens and young adults are getting it. The average age of people who have developed melanoma, a life-threatening form of cancer, has been dropping. And those wonderful "laugh lines" that appear at twenty are beginning to look like serious wrinkles by the time sun-worshipers reach their thirties.

All the attention to and warnings about sun exposure have arisen because of clear-cut evidence that ultraviolet radiation—from the sun or from artificial sources—is virtually the sole cause of skin cancers. And although most skin cancers are not life-threatening, treatment for them can be disfiguring. Such eye conditions as cataracts, macular degeneration, surgery-requiring skin cancers on the eyelid, and melanomas (the deadlier form of skin cancer) can result from unprotected indulgence in the sun.

This risk has always existed, but with the depletion of the ozone layer it has increased. And because fewer people in the past were able to afford vacations under the sun, public and professional awareness was at a far lower level then than it is now.

Ultraviolet Radiation

Although it lies some 93 million miles away from the earth, the sun is the source of all energy on our planet. Life as we know it couldn't have evolved or been sustained without this energy. No wonder many societies have worshiped the sun; they recognized their debt to the sun even before they understood the scientific principles of photosynthesis and the chains of development through which our natural fuels can be traced to the sun.

The center around which the earth and the other planets of the solar system revolve, the sun is a sizzling ball with a mass 332,000 times greater than and a mean density about ¼ that of the earth. It is so hot that its component elements remain completely gaseous. The temperature of its surface is close to 10,000°F (5,500°C), and its interior is even hotter. The energy that comes to earth from the sun is emitted as radiation of various wavelengths, referred to as the *electromagnetic spectrum*. Included in this spectrum are radio waves, X rays, infrared rays, visible light, and ultraviolet radiation (UVR).

Infrared radiation, which we experience as heat, represents 45 percent of the total energy; another 49 percent of the total energy reaching the earth falls into the visible light spectrum, which we perceive as colors. Ultraviolet radiation represents 6 percent of the total energy reaching the earth, and although we don't see it directly, it is strong enough to induce photochemical reactions and to penetrate the skin. Responsible for both immediate and long-term damage to the skin, UVR eventually causes the skin to sag and wrinkle. In short, it can give us anything from an attractive tan to a fiery sunburn, can cause wrinkles and "sun spots," and ultimately can give us cancer. Ultraviolet radiation stimulates certain cells called *melanocytes* to produce a brown pigment called *melanin*. Melanin acts as a natural defense mechanism to UVR exposure and gives skin the tanned look sought by so many. If for some reason we are especially photosensitive (naturally, from an illness, or because of medication), ultraviolet radiation can cause immediate serious damage.

Most of us are aware that the sun is hottest at midday and that, the nearer to the equator we are, the stronger it is. This has to do with the position of the sun in the sky; when the sun is directly overhead, its rays reach us vertically rather than at an angle, minimizing the distance they must travel through the earth's protective atmosphere before striking us. Seasonal changes also affect the ozone layer: where and when it is thinnest, the sun's rays are strongest. Altitude and surrounding terrain also influence the amount of UVR we receive. Snow reflects the sun even more effectively than sand and water. The potential for damage is greater at high altitudes than near sea level, because less atmospheric filtration occurs. Clouds and pollution may obstruct some UVR, but they do not prevent dangerous levels of it from reaching us. Moreover, the ultraviolet radiation from even the newest, most modern tanning parlors is unsafe, too, as will be discussed fully in Part Two.

Three types of UVR are emitted from the sun. The two with which we are concerned are UV-A and UV-B. UV-C is highly toxic to human, plant, and animal life, but fortunately it is absorbed by the ozone layer and by the rest of the earth's atmosphere before it can reach the earth. UV-B, which represents 0.5 percent of the total energy that reaches the earth, can penetrate the top two regions of the skin. It is responsible for redness and burning and can cause immediate damage to the skin. It is more dangerous than UV-A and is recognized as a direct cause of major skin and eye problems, as well as sunburning and tanning. Although UV-A is a much lower intensity than UV-B, it can penetrate the third region of the skin, the dermis. And since UV-A represents 5.5 percent of the total energy reaching us, its potential for damage is great.

Scientists have found that UV-B wavelengths are quite sensitive to small changes in atmospheric ozone concentrations. Consequently, increased levels of UV-B (as well as UV-A) are now reaching the earth as a result of ongoing depletion of the ozone layer high up in the stratosphere. For this reason, even if you spend no more unprotected time in the sun than your parents did, your chances of developing age-damaged skin or cancer are far greater than theirs were when they were your age.

The Earth's Fragile Ozone Layer

Ozone is a form of pure oxygen. A layer of ozone blankets the upper atmosphere, where the atmospheric density is extremely low. Over 99 percent of the atmosphere lies beneath the ozone layer. Ozone is produced when ultraviolet radiation from the sun breaks up normal 2-atom molecules of free oxygen gas and causes them to re-form as 3-atom molecules. O_3 or ozone in the upper atmosphere subsequently traps ultraviolet rays from the sun, thus protecting life on earth from the most dangerous forms of UVR. The risks reduced by this action include skin cancer in humans, damage to marine life, and smaller crop yields. The layer is quite fragile; if all the ozone molecules were compacted into a continuous thin layer, it would be less than 1 inch thick.

Ozone also forms in the lower atmosphere. Exhausts from cars and factories react with radiation from the sun to make ozone. Breathing too much ozone can be dangerous, as joggers and others may find if they inhale too much ozone-polluted air on hot smoggy days.

Until this century, the ozone layer in the stratosphere had remained balanced for billions of years. And because the amount of UV radiation present in the sunlight striking the earth depends on the concentration of ozone, this too remained constant. Plants and animals (including humans) have evolved and lived under that stable amount of untraviolet radiation. Now all of this is changing.

Back in the 1920s, chlorofluorocarbons (CFCs) were first synthesized. These chemicals, composed of chlorine, fluorine, and carbon atoms, do not combine easily with other substances. Because they vaporize at low temperatures, they work well as coolants in refrigerators and air-conditioners and as aerosol propellants in various types of spray cans. They are also good insulators and are widely used in plastic foam materials. They are simple and inexpensive to manufacture.

But in the mid-1970s it was discovered that CFCs float upward a great distance, ultimately reaching ozone molecules in the upper atmosphere. Solar radiation releases the chlorine in the CFCs, which in turn breaks apart the ozone molecules, which then reform as regular molecules of oxygen gas (O_2). In response to scientific concern about the ozone layer, the use of CFCs in spray cans was reduced 60 percent between 1974 and 1978. In 1978, nonessential aerosols of CFCs were banned in the United States, Canada, and Scandinavia. However, the chemicals continued to be produced and used in other ways; and in the rest of the world, CFCs continued to be used in aerosol cans. Overall, production of CFCs increased.

In 1985 a shocking discovery was announced. British scientists had found a hole in the ozone layer, centered over Antarctica. This hole appears every spring, but when the winds change for the rest of the year, the hole seems to reclose. Still, in 1987, ozone levels across the Southern Hemisphere were noted to be down 5 percent over the levels at which they had previously remained stable. Scientists have increased their warnings that the continued manufacture and use of products that contain CFCs pose a major threat to life on the planet, but a total worldwide ban has not yet gone into effect.

What does this mean for us? Even if no more CFCs are released, those already released are likely to remain in the atmosphere for another 100 years. Adverse affects on plant and animal life are almost certain to occur. The sun's rays are now and will remain stronger and more dangerous than they were in previous generations. According to the Skin Cancer Foundation, for each 1 percent drop in stratospheric ozone, there is a 3 to 6 percent increase in nonmelanoma skin cancers and in all likelihood a significant increase in malignant melanoma, too. Increased ultraviolet radiation (particularly UV-B) also suppresses the immune system in a number of ways. It can influence the onset of herpes simplex virus type 1 (better known as cold sores) and some immune diseases such as systemic and discoid lupus erythematosus. Clearly, the sun actually *does* present greater risks today than it did in the past.

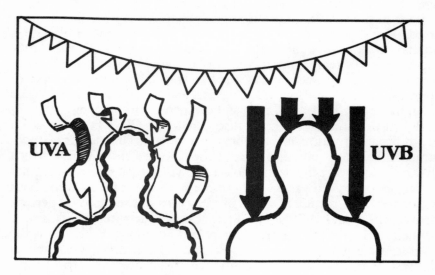

The two types of solar radiation: UVA penetrates deeply to damage your skin's lower layers causing wrinkling and premature aging; UVB ("the sunburn spectrum") is absorbed at the surface, causing burning and peeling.

In May of 1989, a committee was convened by the National Institutes of Health to study sunlight's impact on the skin; it concluded that no type or degree of tanning is safe. The fourteen-member committee said that exposure to ultraviolet radiation from natural sunlight and artificial sources is increasing substantially and that such prolonged exposure causes wrinkles and increases the risk of skin cancer. A report on a study conducted jointly by Kaiser Permanente (a health insurance program) and the National Cancer Institute appeared in the October 23, 1989, issue of the prestigious *Journal of the American Medical Association*. Their findings: two forms of skin cancer—squamous cell skin carcinoma and malignant melanoma—increased between threefold and fourfold over the period from 1960 to 1987. "Both malignancies are considerably more common in this population than we expected based on previous reports from the general population," the study said. "We may be seeing the result of a widespread change in lifestyle, with the increase perhaps related to greater outdoor activity and the use of clothing that offers less sun protection."

Dermatologists have been telling us that for many years, but now it's official.

2

The Skin: How It Reacts to the Sun

We tend to think of our skin as the part of us that is most visible, and indeed it is. Paradoxically, the same people who spend fortunes on cosmetics and even plastic surgery in hopes of having beautiful skin are often the ones who recklessly bask in the sun, trying to achieve a glowing tan.

The skin is the body's largest organ. It protects the internal organs, helps prevent dehydration, and aids in disposing of bodily wastes. The skin differs from other body organs in that worn-out and dead cells are continually (and automatically) shed and regenerated. But don't be misled. Even though your suntan fades as older cells are shed, damage still occurs because the ultraviolet rays of the sun penetrate beyond your skin's visible portion or epidermis.

Tough but supple tissue, the skin is composed of several discrete layers of cells. The topmost of these is called the *stratum corneum or horny layer*. The end product of the maturing cells in this horny layer is keratin, a fibrous protein whose concentration is greatest in parts of the body that are subject to abrasion, such as the palms of the hands and the soles of the feet. It is thinnest in areas such as behind the ear.

The epidermis serves as a barrier to outside elements and bacteria, maintains body temperatures, keeps us from losing body fluids, and prevents us from becoming waterlogged each time we step into the shower or out in the rain. However, this barrier isn't flawless: poisons and ultraviolet radiation can penetrate it, and some medications have been formulated specifically to be absorbed through the skin. Certain conditions such as eczema, psoriasis, or even severe chappedness can cause the skin to lose resiliency; and cuts and other openings in skin can disturb the normal skin barrier, allowing bacteria to enter the body.

Under the stratum corneum lies the *stratum spinosum,* sometimes called the *prickle cell layer.* Here can be found the fast-growing squamous cells that have matured and moved upward from the lowest layer, the *stratum germinativum,* better known as the *basal layer.* Approximately one out of every six cells in the basal layer is a melanocyte, which produces melanin. The amount and the compactness of the arrangement of melanin normally produced are genetically determined: darker-skinned people produce and thus have more melanin than fair-skinned people, and their melanin is distributed more densely. Ultraviolet radiation, from the sun or from tanning devices (as described in chapter 4), stimulates production of melanin, resulting in suntan. Melanin also offers some protection against ultraviolet radiation, which is why fair-skinned people exposed to the sun burn faster and with more damaging results.

Concealed from view beneath the epidermis is the dermis. It contains blood vessels, glands, nerve endings, and connective tissue consisting of elastic and collagen fibers. Also situated in this layer are the Langerhans cells, part of the immune system, whose function is to fight off invasions of foreign substances such as bacteria, viruses, and allergens. The elastic tissues of the dermis are altered with age, as they begin to break down and lose elasticity. The fibers then stiffen, and the skin begins to wrinkle and sag. Genetics play a role in susceptibility, but even the best hereditary support can be offset through excessive exposure to ultraviolet radiation.

Perhaps you are wondering whether collagen or something else can be applied to the face to reach the fibers of the dermis and prevent the skin from appearing to age. Many cosmetic companies in the past have claimed that their products can do this, saying they could reverse or prevent wrinkling and sagging. But so far only Retin-A—a drug originally used to treat acne and available only by prescription (and discussed extensively in Part Three)—has been demonstrated to do this successfully.

Beneath the dermis lies the *subcutis,* also know as the *subcutaneous fatty tissue.* Hair follicles, oil glands, and sweat glands pass through this fatty layer and all the way to the epidermis. These glands aid in maintaining body temperature and in holding moisture in the skin, and this in turn makes skin soft and supple.

Over the years the quantity of fatty tissue diminishes, which explains why older people are often beset with skin injuries and sensitivity to cold. The skin generally becomes thinner, drier, and less resilient. Old and damaged cells can no longer regenerate as fast as they once did. Genetics, diet, and environment are factors that contribute to this timetable, but the sun is the worst enemy your skin can have. In addition to protecting yourself from the sun, you can do other things to keep your skin healthy. These steps will be explored fully in Part Two.

Benefits of the Sun

Notwithstanding all the dangers posed by the sun, some (but not too many) benefits may be derived from sun exposure. The warmth feels good: it can actually lift your mood. I'm writing this on the first sunny day in almost a week, and I find my spirits rising as I look out of the window and see the sun glistening on the treetops.

The Sun and Vitamin D

Sunlight manufactures vitamin D in the skin, and the vitamin is then absorbed by the body. The main function of vitamin D, which is also found in dairy products and in other fortified foods, is to bring about absorption of calcium from the intestinal tract; it is thus essential for the healthy development and growth of bones. Children who do not receive any vitamin D from the sun or in their foods are at risk of developing rickets—a condition in which bones soften and bow, and normal growth is imparied.

In the absence of any unusual medical condition, brief exposure to sunlight on a regular basis anywhere on the body is sufficient to produce an adequate amount of dietary vitamin D. When this is not possible a vitamin D supplement (available in many multivitamins) can be used to obtain the same protection.

There have been some reported concerns about the health of older people whose diets are not rich in vitamin D and who either do not get any sunshine or use sunscreens on all exposed areas of their bodies. In addition, the skin's capacity to produce vitamin D diminishes with aging, which can result in weakened bones and fractures among members of this already vulnerable age group. However, most physicians weighing the risk of skin cancer from sun against the potential of vitamin D deficiency still recommend that a sunscreen be used. Their advice is for older people to adopt a diet of vitamin-D-rich dairy foods or fatty fish, and/or a vitamin D supplement to aid in attaining the Recommended Daily Allowance (RDA) of 400 IUs. They also warn individuals from this population that, just as *too* much sun is dangerous, too much vitamin D can be toxic.

Seasonal Affective Disorder

Sunlight is a morale booster for us all, but for people who suffer from seasonal affective disorder (SAD) it seems to be essential. SAD is a disturbance of mood and behavior that actually resembles certain seasonal changes seen in some lower mammals. People who suffer from this condition experience a depression in the winter, usually starting in early fall and continuing to worsen as the winter progresses. The depressed feelings begin to decrease when the days get longer and warmer in the spring. Symptoms include sadness, anxiety, irritability, decreased physical activity, increased (or sometimes decreased) appetite, carbohydrate craving, weight gain (or sometimes loss), extreme tiredness and need for more sleep, decreased sexual energy, premenstrual symptoms, and difficulties trying to work. Almost all SAD sufferers experience problems with interpersonal relationships during the winter months. Although it is much more common in women than in men, SAD also afflicts men and children. Most often, SAD begins in a person's twenties or thirties.

Specific treatments for this condition exist for people whose doctors have ruled out other psychiatric problems, for whom nothing else is occurring in their lives that could be responsible for the depression, and who have had the problem for at least two fall-winters *and* are fine during the summers. Antidepressant medications may work for some sufferers, but it may not be physiologically desirable for some individuals, and others may simply not want to use them. For these sufferers of SAD, a therapy that makes use of all the wave frequencies present in sunlight is very successful.

The treatment involves regular exposure to full-spectrum bright artificial light of a higher intensity than is usually present in either the home or the workplace. A light fixture that can hold four 40-watt tubes of full-spectrum bright artificial light produces an intensity of light that is anywhere from five to ten times brighter than typical room light. Depending on when the person with SAD experiences his or her symptoms, the physician may recommend using this light therapy in the morning or in the evening, usually for about two hours. This kind of lighting system can be used at home, and those for whom the therapy is successful usually experience a mood change in a matter of days.

SAD isn't treated by exposure to the sun, but it is treated with light that mimics sunlight's effects on a person's visual system, without the danger posed by ultraviolet radiation. It must be noted, however, that this therapy should not be undertaken by a do-it-yourselfer in the absence of professional guidance. If you believe you suffer from SAD, see your family physician, who will probably recommend a psychiatrist familiar with this treatment.

If you just seem to have a better disposition on bright and sunny days, you're not alone. Most of us are cheered by sunshine and/or light. On dark and dreary days, put some extra lights on at home or in the office; wear a bright tie or blouse; surround yourself with some upheat pictures, flowers, or music; and do try to get out for a while on sunny days. Later we'll talk about how you can enjoy the great outdoors without worrying about sun damage.

Treatment of Psoriasis and Alopecia Areata

Some skin disorders are actually treated with artificial "sunshine"—that is, ultraviolet light. Psoriasis is such a disorder. A chronic, noncontagious skin condition that tends to run in some families, it is characterized by red scaly patches covered by thick, silver-gray scales. The cause of the condition is not known, and although psoriasis may sometimes look a little like eczema, it is not a related condition. While stress or physical illness can generate outbreaks, this is not the cause. Psoriasis results from a rapid turnover of epidermal cells that do not mature properly. The immature cells pile up, causing lesions or patches. Since skin usually takes a month to renew itself, most of us aren't aware of this shedding, but in someone with psoriasis the renewal of the top layer of skin occurs so quickly that layers of dead skin just accumulate, prompting itchiness or even painful cracklike sores. Psoriasis can affect any area on the body, but generally it appears on the hands, elbows, knees, legs, nails, genital areas, or scalp. It can occur at any time in life from infancy to old age. A number of people report that their symptoms improve in the summer and get worse during the winter, when there is little exposure to sunlight. Interestingly, psoriasis seldom occurs on the face, where sunlight exposure is likely to occur throughout the year.

Most people who have psoriasis can be treated by a variety of effective drugs. But these medications are sometimes ineffective in treating severe and very disfiguring cases of psoriasis.

One therapy that works well for many psoriasis sufferers is exposure to artificial ultraviolet-B (UV-B) light, sometimes in "combination with applications of coal tar. Generally, a dermatologist (a physician who treats diseases of the skin, hair, and nails) recommends twenty-five treatments under a special therapeutic UV-B light considerably stronger than sunlight.

Are psoriasis sufferers who have been treated with this UV-B treatment at greater risk of skin cancer? Studies are inconclusive, although some indications suggest that such patients are far more likely to develop skin cancers than are patients with psoriasis who were not treated with UV-B therapy. The Skin Cancer Foundation states that the risk may be considerably higher than is reflected in some studies, given that it may take many years of exposure to UVR before skin cancer develops. The foundation recommends that patients being treated with UV-B place a lightweight shield, such as a pillowcase, over their head if arms or legs are being treated, and that they even wear gloves to protect hands. The foundation also emphasizes that tanning salons are no substitute for therapeutic ultraviolet treatment. Tanning salons are discussed in chapter 3.

Some patients are treated with PUVA, which makes use of a light-sensitizing medication called *Psoralen* that is applied topically (on the surface of the affected area), taken internally, or in some cases put into bathwater. Then the patient is placed under a therapeutic dose of ultraviolet-A (UV-A) light. According to the Skin Cancer Foundation, the skin cancer risk for patients who receive PUVA treatments is in the range of 10 to 15 percent, so the foundation recommends that, unless the psoriasis is very extensive, UV-B be tried first. PUVA treatment, like the UV-B treatment discussed earlier, is not to be confused with tanning salons, or home "sunlamps." It must be administered under meticulous medical supervision, and care must be taken during the treatment to protect the eyes. PUVA is used both for stubborn cases of psoriasis and for alopecia areata, a disease in which the body forms antibodies against some of the hair follicles. Small, smooth, round, or oval patches of baldness appear on the scalp or beard of individuals with this condition. Sometimes alopecia areata clears up spontaneously. But when it doesn't, PUVA may be utilized.

At one time people thought that many health benefits could be derived from the sun, and although we know better now, at some unconscious level we do tend to think that the sun is good for us. Yet in just these few pages we have covered all the known health benefits of the sun and/or ultraviolet radiation. Still, we ought not minimize the pleasure to be obtained from basking in the warmth of the sun. So, in order to enjoy it but still protect ourselves, let us investigate exactly what the sun can do to our skin.

Some People Are Just More Likely to Have Problems with the Sun

I was a teenager just after World War II, and I remember two sisters who belonged to our beach club. They had very blonde hair, pale skin, and blue eyes. The older sister, whom I shall call Louise, used to swim and linger in the sun with all the other kids, despite some rather nasty sunburns; but her younger sister, whom I will call Kate, seemed like a daytime recluse in the summer. She would keep to the shade, wear a big hat and sunglasses, and only venture out in the sun when it was absolutely necessary. The rest of the kids—including me—thought she was a bit weird.

But now I know better. For one thing, I ran into Kate one day at a concert. I recognized her immediately: she had hardly changed. Her skin looked young and beautiful, and even with my glasses on I couldn't see any wrinkles. We caught up on each other's lives, and she told me that Louise had moved to Arizona. I told her I was in the midst of researching this book, hoping that she might tell me how her sister had fared from her years in the sun.

"Louise still loves the sun," said Kate, "but she's paid a high price for it. She's had a few basal cell cancers removed and also had dermabrasion and a chemical peel just to eliminate wrinkles. So now, she *does* stay out of the sun."

I asked Kate why she had had the foresight to hide from the sun in those days before we really knew the dangers and prior to the availability of effective sunscreens. She responded, "You know my whole family was very fair-skinned, and I remember my grandmother looked older than anyone else's grandmother. She had some awful little wartlike pink things on her face. I didn't know it then, but I guess it was kind of a precancer. Anyway, Grandma told me that from the time she was a little girl in Minnesota she had spent hours in the sun, summers and winters, and she kept doing that after she grew up. She said she thought that had caused her skin to change the way it had. I guess that scared me. Anyway, I'm glad I got the message, even if I didn't have too much fun those summers."

All of that hiding from the sun and not having much fun with the rest of us during the day doesn't seem to have put too much of a damper on Kate's subsequent lifestyle. She's a real-estate broker, has been married to the same man for over thirty years, and has two children. We showed each other pictures of our children and young grandchildren, and Kate said, "My daughter Julia thought I was a bit of a character, too, when she was growing up; but we avoided beaches and vacationed at lakeside areas where there were plenty of trees for me to sit under. Julia wasn't fair like me, so like most of the mothers I didn't take any special precautions. But see: here's Julia's little girl—fairer than I was."

Indeed, Heather looked like a little Scandinavian princess. "Thank goodness they make all those wonderful sunscreens now so she can have fun in the sun without this crazy grandmother hovering over her," Kate laughingly told me.

Right you are, Kate! Heather and her friends and their moms and dads and grandparents can all enjoy being outdoors, summer and winter, if they take sensible precautions. Knowing your susceptibility to skin damage from the sun is a starter.

Skin Types as a Predictor of Damage from the Sun

In many ways, Kate was ahead of her time, although most very fair-skinned people know that they usually burn rather than get a beautiful tan. Researchers today are able to confirm that people with fair skin, red or light hair color, light eye color, and freckles are likely to burn severely and, even if they do eventually tan, suffer cumulative damage.

The concept of skin typing came into being in the mid-1970s, when studies were done under careful laboratory conditions to categorize and measure a person's skin response to sunlight. The extent of a person's sensitivity to ultraviolet radiation is measured as the minimal erythema (sunburn) dose of UVR that provokes even the slightest perceptible sunburn in that person's skin. Referred to as an *MED value,* this measurement bears a strong (though not absolute) relationship to skin type.

Why is it that some types of skin seem to burn more easily than others? Quite simply, it has to do with the amount of melanin in the skin: the more melanin, the more protection against UVR damage. As was mentioned earlier, melanin, a brown pigment, is produced by epidermal cells called *melanocytes.* Everyone, from fair-skinned people to black-skinned people, has the same number of melanocytes. However, the rate of production of melanin in your skin is determined by the stimulation it receives, as well as by your genes. Thus, fair-skinned people such as Kate and Louise, who have less melanin in place from the start, also have melanocytes that don't respond to the sun by producing a nice all-over tan; instead they burn. If they foolishly persist in sunning themselves, they may develop a tan by the end of the summer, but the damage to their skin is accumulating. Some people almost as fair as Kate and Louise may be able to tan more easily, and some people with much darker skin tones may burn easily; generally, however, the darker the skin, the greater the protection from ultraviolet radiation.

Dermatologists recommend that you learn your skin type, because you can use this guide as a way of safeguarding yourself from the effects of the sun. Although the accompanying chart does not discuss ethnic groups, generally those with Type 1 or 2 skin are of Celtic,

Scandinavian, or North European descent. Type 3, 4, and 5 typically include descendents of Italians, Spaniards, and Greeks; Type 5 descendents of Asians and many Hispanics; and Type 6 descendents of Black Africans. But since ethnic groups have merged over the years, many Africans (and Asian-Americans) have light skin, and some North Europeans are quite dark.

People who are least sensitive to the sun (skin types of the higher numbers) have the greatest concentration of melanin in their dermis. These pigments, which are formed in the basal layer of the skin, move up to the stratum corneum in response to ultraviolet radiation, and this results in a tanned appearance. People with the greatest sensitivity to the sun (skin types of the lower numbers) have a lower concentra-

Skin Types and Skin Reactions to Ultraviolet Radiation

Skin Type	Reaction to Sun	Examples
Type I	Always burns, sometimes painfully; seldom or never tans; peels; extremely sensitive to UVR	People with fair skin, blue or sometimes brown eyes, freckles, blonde or red hair
Type II	Usually burns, sometimes painfully; sometimes tans, but not very much; may peel; very sensitive to UVR	People with fair skin, red, blonde, or brown hair, and blue, hazel, or brown eyes
Type III	Burns moderately; tans gradually; sensitive to UVR	Average Caucasian
Type IV	Seldom burns; tans easily and reacts with almost immediate darkening of skin (IPD: Immediate Pigment Darkening); moderately sensitive to UVR.	People with white, olive, or light brown skin, dark brown hair, and dark eyes
Type V	Almost never burns; tans easily and considerably; IPD reaction; minimally sensitive to UVR	Brown-skinned people, often of Asian or Indian descent
Type VI	Never burns, but tans greatly; IPD reaction; not sensitive to UVR	African-Americans

tion of melanin in their dermis, which is why they burn rather than tan.

Some dermatologists believe that relying on this chart may give you a false sense of security. They note that striking individual differences occur, and they point out that someone with dark skin and hair may still be very vulnerable. They suggest that you try to recall whether some time in the past you tanned or burned after a 45-minute exposure at noon on a hot summer day—without sunscreens. Don't try it now, but think back to those days before you were cautious and sensible.

If you are one of the lucky people who tans but doesn't burn, you do have more protection than your fair-skinned friends from that noon-day sun. But *only* about as much as if you were wearing a Sun Protection Factor (SPF) sunscreen of 2 or 3. And if you have developed a gradual deep tan, that offers you at most the equivalent of an SPF of 4. That's not very much, considering that the Skin Cancer Foundation recommends that everyone use a sunscreen with an SPF of 15 or higher.

"I'll be careful and just tan slowly," says my young friend Janet. She has typical, average Type 3 skin and looks beautiful all year long; but by mid-July her golden tan, dark brown hair, bright red lipstick, and smashing white pantsuit definitely make heads turn. Janet isn't as likely as a very fair-skinned person to run into the troubles that have beset Louise, but she is gambling with the possibility of developing a number of problems including skin cancer. Why? The melanin in her skin is still insufficient to protect the deeper layers of the skin from absorbing the sun's rays. Sandra, my dark-skinned African-American friend, is on much safer ground. Absorption of UVR by her epidermis is greater than Janet's, so approximately five times less ultraviolet radiation reaches her dermis than reaches that of the average Caucasian. Although skin cancer is not as common in black-skinned people as in lighter-skinned individuals, they are not totally immune to it and to other problems emanating from the sun. In Chapter 4, the subject of black skin is discussed in more depth.

Extreme Reactions to Ultraviolet Radiation

Certain people are at special risk of damage from UVR. They were born with partial or total lack of melanin pigment in their body (a condition called *albinism)*, and they are prone to severe sunburn, skin inflammations or rash, and skin cancer—all resulting from *any* exposure to ultraviolet radiation. Total albinos have pale skin, white hair, and pink eyes, and their skin and eyes have an abnormal sensitivity to light. Albinism is represented in all ethnic groups.

People suffering from vitiligo, a skin disease that can develop at any age, have irregular patches of various sizes that are totally lacking in pigment. Often these patches have unusually dark borders. The cause of vitiligo is not known, but it may be related to other autoimmune diseases in which the body acts against some of its own cells (in this case, against melanocytes responsible for producing melanin). These unpigmented patches may burn after only brief exposure to the sun; thus extreme care must be taken by those who have vitiligo.

A number of other conditions are often activated, prompted, or exacerbated by sunlight. Among them are most types of acne, herpes simplex, psoriasis, and viral infections of the skin. Contrary to the popular belief that "a little suntan" is good for these conditions, people who have them are likely to find that their skin troubles increase after exposure to sun. Eczema may be an exception: some people say that the sun actually improves it, but others find that the sun aggravates the condition. True, a nice tan will mask skin imperfections, but products are available that cover imperfections—whether an innocuous rash or a deep and large scar—similarly, with no health risk.

People who have discoid lupus erythematosus (DLE) or systemic lupus erythematosus (SLE) react very poorly to the sun. The former is a chronic, recurrent disease, primarily of the skin, with a characteristic red, scaly, butterflylike pattern covering the cheeks and bridge of the nose; it can also occur on other parts of the body. The latter is also a chronic disease, but it is inflammatory and can affect many systems of the body. One-third to one-half of all people with lupus are photosensitive, which means that they are extremely sensitive to sunlight or any form of ultraviolet radiation. In these people, severe sunburn is only one possible consequence of sun exposure: they may experience anything from a minor flare-up of symptoms to a serious exacerbation of their disease requiring intensive medical attention.

Almost 10 percent of otherwise healthy people are affected by a disorder called polymorphous light eruption (PMLE). Usually before the age of thirty, these individuals exhibit an abnormal response to the light from UV-A and UV-B. Those affected are most often fair-skinned women, and their symptoms include recurrent sunburns, raised skin lesions, tiny blisters, and other skin eruptions.

A number of people suffer solar urticaria, a photosensitive reaction that develops within minutes of exposure to sunlight or even artificial light sources. Although rare, it can be severe in its eruptions and frequency.

Also known to cause photosensitivity in some people are various inherited disorders in which the body abnormally produces certain parts of the hemoglobin molecule located in the red blood cells. Such disorders, known under the general term of *porphyrias,* range from mild to rather serious. Sufferers are extremely sensitive to UVR because these substances affect their bodies much as do the photosensitive drugs discussed in the next section.

Xeroderma pigmentosa is an extremely rare genetic disorder characterized by sun sensitivity and an inability to repair ultraviolet-damaged DNA. Individuals who have it develop skin cancer at a frequency more than 1,000 times that of the general population.

Chemical Photosensitivity

The term *chemical photosensitivity* refers to adverse skin reactions resulting from exposure to both UVR and any of various chemicals. For instance, some people will suffer skin rashes, severe sunburn, or hives if they go out in sunlight following contact with insecticides or the coal tar extracts used in asphalt and roofing materials. Certain medications taken internally or applied topically to the skin can cause similar reactions. Some common plants are similarly implicated: limes, lemons, garden-variety parsnip, celery, fennel, dill, garden carrots, and buttercups, among others.

Photosensitive reactions vary not only with the contributing chemicals, but somewhat among people. For instance, assorted perfumes, colognes, shaving products, and deodorants contain ingredients that absorb light into the skin of some individuals, causing a bad sunburn or rash where the substance has been applied. Meanwhile, someone else using the same product may have no problem at all.

Warnings are printed on the labels of numerous medications that are known photosensitizers. Look for words to the following effect: "This product may cause adverse reaction to ultraviolet rays." Always read any inserts in the medication you take, and consider obtaining a consumer-oriented guide (see the bibliography) to both prescription and nonprescription drugs that you can consult before taking any medication. If you have any doubt about the safety of a medication, or if you know you will be going out in the sun after taking it, discuss the situation with your physician or pharmacist.

Here are some photosensitizers: antibiotics such as the sulfonamides, vibramycin, grisulvin, minocycline, and tetracyline; many antifungal medications; Tolbutamide (orinase) and Chlorpropamide (diabinese), the oral medications taken by diabetics; diuretics including those known as Diuril, Hydrodiuril or HCTZ, and Lasix; antidepressants such as Elavil and Norpramin; tranquilizers including Librium, Thorazine, Haldol, and Navane; Psoralen, which was discussed earlier as a treatment for psoriasis; and birth control pills. Appendix II provides a further listing of phototoxic and photoallergenic compounds.

The list seems almost endless. Medications that contain ingredients from the coal tar group and used for treating eczema and psoriasis, nalalidixic acid prescribed for certain urinary tract infections, and a number of antihistamines are also on the compendium of chemicals that cause photosensitivity. Obviously, the medications you take internally may cause an adverse skin reaction wherever you are exposed to UVR, but cosmetics or medications applied to the skin are likely to cause problems only in that area.

Many of the drugs involved in chemotherapy to treat cancer are photosensitizers. Discuss this subject with your doctor or nurse if you are receiving chemotherapy.

In some instances, the adverse response to the sun may occur almost immediately; in others, no symptoms appear until hours or even days after exposure. My friend Sarah wondered why she always developed a miserable eczema-like rash every time she took a winter vacation, despite never having problems in the summer when she played tennis or golf near her home. Her dermatologist was a good medical detective: she discovered that Sarah always took a diuretic before flying because she, like many people, has a tendency to develop swollen ankles during airplane flights. Sarah's diuretic made her photosensitive; but her husband, who takes one regularly for his high blood pressure, never gets into trouble in the sun. (For several years, he has been careful to wear a sunscreen with an SPF of more than 15 and a golf hat to cover his thinning hair before he goes outside.) People who become photosensitive after exposure to some chemicals may, like Sarah, develop a rash, or they may suffer a severe sunburn.

Ouch! A Sunburn Hurts

Who is likely to get sunburned? Anyone exposed to intense UVR may, but people with the sensitive Type 1 or 2 skin are at the greatest risk because their skin has the lowest concentration of protective melanin in the dermis.

The very young and the elderly are particularly prone to injury from the sun. Young people often have lighter skin than they will have in later years, and unless they are well instructed and motivated in sun protection techniques (discussed in chapter 5), they are likely to ignore the danger. As adults age, their skin becomes thinner and they may have fewer melanocytes, so they are more vulnerable to burning, too.

Anyone who has been exposed to the sun on a gradual basis and built up a tan is less likely to burn. This is because the sun's rays speed up mitosis of the epidermal cells, causing thickening of the stratum corneum in four to seven days, which in turn renders the skin less penetrable to UVR. But dermatologists remind us that just because you don't burn doesn't mean the sun is not doing damage. It is.

If you have ever had a severe or even moderately uncomfortable sunburn, you probably remember just what it felt like. Your skin turned pink or even scarlet, and there may have been some mild swelling. Later in the evening—perhaps just as you were trying to get to sleep, or maybe the next day—your skin may have turned even brighter red, with considerable attendant swelling or blistering. Anything (including water) touching the skin made you want to scream in pain. Perhaps you had strap marks where a bathing suit's covering ended, but if you were wearing a lightweight cotton covering, some of the sunlight may have penetrated to render the line between the unburned and sunburned areas almost unidentifiable. Some areas of the skin are more sensitive than others, and naturally any sunburned area that you had to cover before going out in public bothered you the most. Your skin may have felt tender, warm, and tight, and the sunburn probably itched. It may have been painful, but the worst was probably over within 24 hours. If you suffered an extremely severe sunburn (sometimes called *sun poisoning*), however, you might have become nauseated, sustained chills and fever, and even suffered from tachycardia (accelerated heart rate) in addition to experiencing blistering and peeling.

The explanation for this sunburn process is still not fully understood, but experts believe that, when the epidermis is damaged by UVR, the dead epidermal cells become unevenly distributed, and the body responds by releasing various chemical substances that precipitate skin inflammation. Among these substances are prostaglandins, which may widen the small blood vessels of the skin, causing the redness. As the blood supply to the burnt area increases, tissue fluid and white blood cells collect there and cause swelling. Water is lost through the skin, and you may actually become dehydrated.

Sunburn on lips can be especially painful. Lifeguards know this, so they cover their lips with a total sunblock like thick zinc oxide. People who are fair-skinned, have protruding lips, or breathe through their mouths and habitually keep their lips parted are especially vulnerable to severe sunburn there, sometimes resulting in dreadful sores.

Sunburns eventually heal without any scars, unless an infection develops because damage prevented tissue from protecting itself against bacteria. Mild sunburns can usually be treated with an assortment of nonprescription remedies that are applied to the skin; some are in lotion form, and others are sprays. If symptoms persist, medical attention should be sought.

The best way to avoid sunburn and the accompanying discomfort and damage to skin is to prevent it by using sunscreen and wearing protective clothing whenever you are exposed to ultraviolet radiation. In Part Two, you will learn different ways to protect yourself from UVR and still enjoy outdoor life, and in Part Three you'll find out how to treat sunburn.

Sunstroke

Sunstroke or heatstroke can happen to anyone—a child, an old person, an athlete, or anyone else who has allowed his or her body temperature to rise to a dangerously high level. Unlike heat exhaustion, which usually responds to rest and replacement of body fluids and salts, heatstroke is a medical emergency that can be fatal.

Heatstroke can happen in the shade or in an overheated house, but frequently it is the result of too much sun. The symptoms are very hot, dry skin and no sweating, along with a body temperature of 104°F or higher, weakness, dizziness, rapid breathing, nausea, and sometimes mental confusion or unconsciousness that may occur suddenly and dramatically.

First aid for heatstroke consists of cooling the person quickly by applying an ice bag or crushed ice, by wrapping the person in wet sheets, or even by hosing the person down with cold water. Then get the victim to an emergency room, or call the local medics!

It's clear that, aside from the long-term ravages caused by the sun (some of which we will discuss later), sunstroke or heatstroke are very real hazards.

Altitudes, Latitudes, Summer, Winter, Beach, and Sports

The nearer to the equator you are, the stronger the UVR is. Anyone who has ever taken a Caribbean or Mexican vacation and compared the sun there to summers in Maine can attest to that. Consequently, we are more likely to beware of getting a blistering or painful sunburn from a vacation on the islands or from a clear day at our hometown beach during midsummer. But a person can get a sunburn while sitting under an umbrella on a cloudy day. Ultraviolet radiation reaches and penetrates your skin even when there is little visible sun, and even in the dead of winter—especially at high altitudes.

For every 1,000 feet of elevation above sea level, ultraviolet light intensifies 4 to 5 percent. Thus, if you are skiing at an altitude of 5,000 feet, you will be exposed to 20 to 25 percent more UVR than will someone sitting around the lodge at sea level.

Many skiers have had their vacations marred by severe cases of sunburn. Some time ago, researchers in India studied 67 student mountaineers during three expeditions. Even though they took some precautions, many of the students suffered sunburn. The greater intensity of ultraviolet radiation at high altitude is due to decreased atmospheric pressure, reduced quantities of ozone and oxygen in the air, and increased reflectance from the surface of the surrounding snow. The combination of these factors increases a person's chance of becoming sunburned.

People who have had herpes on their face are likely to suffer a recurrence of it when they ski. The sun can trigger this reactivation, and (as we have seen) skiers are especially subject to UVR from the sun. However, one scientific study found that use of a protective sunscreen didn't significantly reduce the rate of recurrence of herpes. A possible explanation for this is that the herpes might have been triggered in these skiers by stimulation of facial nerves by wind and cold, as well as by the sun.

The sun also takes its toll on surfers, according to Mark Renneker, MD, a California physician who is also president of the Surfer's Medical Association. He recommends that, since some surfers have practiced the sport for many years, predating the awareness of skin cancer and its prevention, physicians be especially careful in examining such individuals. Surfers are at a high risk for skin damage: water reflects the sun, and anyone who spends a great deal of time on it, whether swimming, surfing, or boating, is subject to the negative effects of the sun.

Other outdoor sports participants are at risk for damage from the sun, as well. For example, studies of female golfers clearly showed a significant difference in the incidence of skin cancer between professionals and amateurs. The professionals were younger than the amateurs and had been playing for fewer years, but they still had more cancers. Why is this? Professionals are more likely than the amateurs to practice or play golf at midday and under other conditions in which sunlight is especially intense, and they usually begin playing golf when they are quite young. Studies suggest that prolonged daily sun exposure may be more important in causing skin cancer than occasional sunburns; that excessive heat, humidity, and wind can have a similar effect. (Professional tournaments are often played under those conditions.) Finally, that exposure to ultraviolet radiation early in life has a major impact on development of skin cancer later in life. Many years ago, a study demonstrated that people who lived their early lives in southern climes had a higher rate of skin cancer than a matched group who grew up in the north. And more recent studies suggest that, starting at midlife, susceptibility to skin cancer may increase because of the body's decreased ability to repair damaged tissues.

The implications of these studies are clear. Those who play—and certainly those who work—outdoors during the hottest, sunniest days or who spend much time surrounded by snow or water need to be especially vigilant.

Photoaging

Photoaging does not allude, as you might think, to the fading and discoloration of old snapshots. Rather, it refers to both obvious and microscopic skin changes that result from years of exposure to ultraviolet radiation. For many years, these changes were simply considered to be an exaggerated or accelerated form of normal aging. But now it is becoming increasingly clear that photoaging is something quite different.

Fifty-year-old sun-worshipers with Type 1 skin may look much older than their chronological age, exhibiting numerous pigmented brown age-spots and skin that is wrinkled, yellowed, dry, and leathery. On the other hand, seventy- and eighty-year-olds who never went out in the sun may have smooth, unwrinkled skin that reveals only some thinning, deepening of lines, and loss of elasticity.

Because years of sun exposure may pass before photoaging begins to take place, people have often attributed their aging look to bad luck. But although most people will have a progressive deepening of normal expression lines and will develop some fine wrinkles over the years, those who have had a great deal of sun exposure will acquire deep wrinkles and a bumpy, leathery-textured skin. Some changes are inevitable, since cell renewal of the epidermis slows down with aging, but serious sunbathers also have a number of precancerous cells in the epidermis. Everyone loses collagen and experiences some breakdown in elastic tissue and blood vessels, but those who have spent hour after hour in the sun suffer a significant diminution in elasticity, a pronounced loss of collagen, and a decrease in blood vessels. It is not unusual to develop telangiectases—a condition in which "broken" blood vessels assume a fishnet appearance on face, neck, or chest. These changes are apparent to the naked eye and under the microscope.

What about people with darkly pigmented skin? Whether Caucasian, Asian, Hispanic, or African, such people have some resistance to the damage caused by the sun. According to some estimates, people with Type 5 or 6 skin may have a ten-year grace period of sun exposure without loss of elasticity. In chapter 4, which focuses on black skin, we will consider this more fully.

Sooner or later, chronic exposure to sun will contribute to photoaging in any person, but the ravages of the sun are far worse for some people than for others. Perhaps you are thirty and have noticed that those laugh lines are setting in deeper; or maybe you just attended your thirty-fifth high-school reunion and realized that you look as old as some of your teachers who spend *their* vacations sight-seeing from buses and touring inside museums, while you sit on the beach. But don't despair. It's never to late to protect your skin from further damage, as we discuss in Part Two. Furthermore, repair for photoaged skin is possible. You'll learn about some of the available options in Part Three.

Solar Lentigines

You've seen solar lentigines (singular: *Lentigo*), even if you didn't know that's what they are called. These brown, flat spots on the backs of hands and on the face look a bit like freckles, but they are usually larger, darker, and less even. Sometimes they are called *liver spots* or *old-age* or *senile freckles,* although they are not freckles and are not associated with the liver.

They appear on people who have had a great deal of exposure to the sun, and although they can be quite unattractive they are neither harmful nor likely to become malignant. A nonphysician, however, may confuse them with malignant melanoma and become needlessly alarmed. Conversely, a person may ignore an early-stage melanoma, imagining that the brown mark is just a solar lentigo. Thus, it is important to consult a physician about any spot that enlarges, thickens, changes, or occurs any time in the lifespan. In chapter 8 we will describe common moles and melanomas.

If you feel that these solar lentigines are unsightly, you can have them removed by electrosurgery or through chemical applications. These techniques will be discussed in Part Three.

In addition to skin-induced aging and solar lentigines, various lesions of the mouth and lips may result from too many sun-filled days.

Actinic or Solar Keratoses

Actinic keratoses—also called *solar keratoses* because they appear almost exclusively on individuals who spend a great deal of time in the sun— begin as pink spots that are smooth and flat or slightly raised above the skin surface, but they eventually become irregular, scaly, and wartlike and turn red or brownish in color. They almost always occur in sun-exposed areas such as the forehead, nose, tips of the ears, upper cheeks, and backs of the hands. People with Type 1 or 2 skin are especially vulnerable to actinic keratoses.

They can be quite unsightly, but of far greater importance is their strong potential for progressing to become squamous cell cancers. For this reason actinic keratoses need to be carefully observed and treated to prevent their further growth. Several effective treatments, all of which offer a cure, are discussed in Part Three.

The Sun's Effect on the Immune System

It's amazing how many myths most of us grew up believing. I always thought that sunlight was a healing force and that a good vacation in the sun, summer or winter, would help fortify me for the school year ahead. But was I ever wrong!

Scientific evidence indicates an association between exposure to ultraviolet radiation and suppression of the immune system. Cancer—and skin cancer in particular—has been closely linked with immunosuppression in a number of situations. For instance, people treated with immunosuppressive chemotherapy drugs for lymphomas appear to be at increased risk for the development of skin cancers. And organ transplant patients, who take medications that suppress their immune system so that they won't reject the new organ, have an increased incidence of cancer development. Stephen E. Ullrich and Margaret L. Kripke of the Department of Immunology at the University of Texas's M. D. Anderson Cancer Center published data on this subject in the 1989 *Journal of the Skin Cancer Foundation*. In discussing kidney transplant patients they say, "There is a preponderance of skin cancers in these patients and most are found on sun-exposed sites of the body. These data suggest that like murine [mouse] skin cancer, the development of human skin cancer may be associated with suppression of the immune response."

How does ultraviolet radiation suppress the immune system? First, let's review how the immune system works. Under normal circumstances, the body recognizes and destroys foreign invaders before they endanger its health. If the body didn't have this ability, minor cuts, infections, and illnesses could be fatal. The foreign invaders, called *antigens,* are recognized by the body, which then mobilizes to attack them. White blood cells attack the bacteria (or other antigens) and stimulate the production of antibodies in the blood plasma. These antibodies then circulate through the bloodstream and attack the antigens. The antibodies continue to circulate after the original invasion has been defeated, and they are able to recognize the same antigens if they ever try to reenter the body. This explains why some childhood illnesses give us lifelong immunity and why vaccination (which makes use of weak antigens to stimulate antibody production) can give your body the same antibody protection as if you had already had the disease in its more virulent form.

Three kinds of cells are important in the immune system: B cells, T cells, and natural killer (NK) cells. *B cells,* manufactured in the bone marrow, produce antibodies that help defend the body against infection or toxic substances. *T cells* are stimulated by antigens to circulate throughout the body. These cells, produced in the thymus gland, are among the larger number of lymphocytes—colorless cells produced in lymphoid organs such as lymph nodes, the spleen, and the thymus.

Natural killer (NK) cells are stimulated by viral infections, possibly through production of interferon—a chemical substance that is itself naturally released by the body in response to viral infections. The natural resistance conferred by NK cells differs from the immunity acquired through previous exposure and is not caused by B or T cells.

Scientists now recognize that anyone with a suppressed or deficient immune system is susceptible to a number of diseases, including cancer. Individuals who already have cancer have low immunity and are especially vulnerable to infections and other illnesses. Although researchers are hard at work trying to find ways to strengthen existing immune systems, it is essential that we avoid anything likely to weaken our immune system.

If (as more and more evidence suggests) excessive exposure to ultraviolet radiation lowers the body's immunity, that in itself should be a good reason to be wary of the sun.

As was noted earlier in this chapter, the skin serves as the main barrier between our body and our environment. All kinds of things brush up against and try to enter our skin: viruses, fungi, bacteria, and chemical and physical carcinogens. The skin is protective not just because it is the body's outer covering but because it possesses a number of properties that collectively permit it to be called an immune organ. The Langerhans cells of the dermis and epidermis are antigen-presenting cells that are capable of communication with T and some non-T lymphocytes.

Although the relationship between skin cancer and exposure to sunlight was noted almost 100 years ago, and although it was demonstrated in the 1920s that ultraviolet radiation can cause skin cancer in mice, understanding of the relationship between ultraviolet radiation and the immune system is far more recent. Basically, transformation of cells by UVR is thought to occur as a result of changes in the nuclear DNA.

Studies in mice indicate that those treated with UVR show an increased incidence of leukemia, lymphoma, and skin cancer, suggesting that UV-induced immunological changes may have great significance for humans. Ullrich and Kripke posed the question "Does UV also suppress the human immune response?" They then described a study in which healthy volunteers were exposed to the radiation generated by a commercial tanning bed. After the volunteers underwent twelve 30-minute exposures, a blood sample was taken from each and an immune profile was done. Sure enough, the immune system's reactivity to certain allergens was depressed, and T cell and

NK cell functions were adversely affected. Similar results were reported after volunteers were exposed to natural sunlight.

Do sun-worshipers, like the mice that were exposed to UVR, have an increased risk of developing such nonskin cancers as leukemia and lymphoma? Is their immune system harmed in such a way that they are vulnerable to numerous minor or serious disorders? The jury is still out, but it is certainly worth considering these possibilities before you take off unprotected for a vacation under the sun.

Photoallergies

A *photoallergy* is defined as a bodily response to some chemical that involves participation of the immune system after exposure to ultraviolet radiation. Photoallergies differ from the phototoxic reactions to chemicals discussed earlier in that, with photoallergic reactions, each time an exposure occurs, the reaction is more severe. Some ingredients in cosmetics (such as fragrances, antibiotic agents, and antifungal agents) and in sunscreens (particularly PABA) have been reported to cause photoallergenic reactions in a number of people. Such reactions can be as simple as a skin rash or as severe as a very uncomfortable eczema-like rash that may scale or crust. Ceasing to use the offending allergen usually eliminates the problem, although often the rash must be treated by a dermatologist with medications that include antihistamines or steroids.

Distinguishing between photosensitivity and photoallergy may be difficult, but it helps determine the most effective treatment. Thus, any rash or skin eruption that occurs and worsens or that fails to clear up when you have removed what you suspect might be the offending cause should be checked by a physician, preferably a dermatologist.

Summary

The skin, our largest organ, serves as a barrier to penetration, but can also be a gateway to the inner organs. Even with the best care, some visible aging of the skin will occur, but the sun hastens and alters this process and is responsible for changes that might never occur if exposure to ultraviolet radiation is kept to a minimum.

The people most vulnerable to skin damage from UVR exposure are those with light skin tones and coloring. Actinic keratoses (areas of skin in a premalignant condition), skin cancers, and malignant melanoma have all been attributed to UVR exposure.

In addition, some people have extreme reactions to UVR. Those who have autoimmune conditions or allergies, are required to take certain medications, or have contact with chemicals are particularly subject to photosensitivity. Evidence is also accumulating that the immune system is compromised by UVR exposure.

Advantages of sun exposure are few: sunlight helps to manufacture vitamin D, which in turn helps to bring about absorption of calcium from the intestinal tract. But proper diet and occasional sunlight can accomplish the same result with minimal risk. People who have seasonal affective disorder (SAD) seem to suffer from lack of sufficient sunlight, but this problem can be treated with artificial (non-UV) light.

Ultraviolet radiation can reach our skin and penetrate it even when we least expect it: in winter as well as in summer, on cloudy days as well as on sunny ones.

Sunlight warms us and lifts our spirits, and we all enjoy it. Learning to be safe in the sun is an attainable goal.

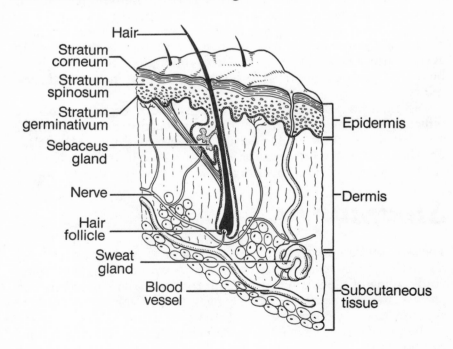

3

Sunless Tanning: Tanning Salons, Tanning Accelerators, and Self-tanners

You've heard the claims: "Indoor tanning: safer than the sun with absolutely no harmful side effects." Entrepreneurs and devotees of this kind of artificial ultraviolet radiation contend that it is safer than a day at the beach or on the ski slopes, and can actually prevent you from the damaging rays to which you will be exposed outdoors.

Questions and Answers About Sunless Tanning

If you've been thinking of getting a tan without spending the time and money on an island vacation, you will want to know more about the safety of these devices. To clear up the confusion, I consulted members of the American Academy of Dermatology, the Skin Cancer Foundation, and the FDA. The question-and-answer section that follows is a synthesis of the reports provided by these experts.

What are sunless tanning devices, and how do they work?
For many years, various artificial sources of ultraviolet radiation have been widely used for tanning in the United States. People could buy single- or double-lamp devices at drug stores and variety stores. Resorts sometimes had a sunroom with overhead sunlamps or other devices that emitted UVR. The ones currently available are usually referred to as *tanning beds* or *booths*. They are clamshell-like Plexiglas units on which the would-be tanner lies; lights from above and below reach the body. At one time these units emitted shortwave ultraviolet radiation (UV-B), but it soon became evident that UV-B was implicated in an increased risk of skin cancer, so these devices now use long-wave ultraviolet light sources (UV-A), which advertisers claim

are safe. However, although these devices may be advertised as producing only UV-A, many of them also emit some UV-B as well.

Where are these tanning devices available?
They are available just about everywhere. Health clubs, beauty salons, barber shops, gas stations, and videotape outlets may have one or more tanning beds; tanning salons can be found in malls and in neighborhood shopping centers across the nation. Home units are also available. Figures obtained from the Food and Drug Administration's Center for Devices and Radiological Health, which has responsibility for regulating the manufacture of these devices, indicate that almost 170,000 home units were sold between 1980 and 1988. Almost 200,000 of the more expensive tanning booths or beds, which are seldom found in homes, were purchased for use in commercial establishments during the same period. The tanning industry association and other business sources estimate that tanning salons are a $1.46 billion per year industry. By the end of 1988, according to a survey of Yellow Pages ads, there were nearly 20,000 tanning salons in the United States.

They have become especially popular near college campuses, where students like to get a headstart on Spring Break. One enterprising young man opened a one-stop business near a large city university where students can drop off dry cleaning, do laundry, get a tan while waiting, and pick up a video and the snacks to go with it.

Who uses tanning beds?
According to a May 1989 report issued by a committee convened by the National Institutes of Health, more than 1 million Americans artificially tan themselves every day. Young executives with no time for a vacation and people on a budget who can't afford a week in the sun in February think tanning beds are great. They feel that they look as well-rested and glowing as their jet-setting neighbors. In 1986, the American Academy of Dermatology estimated that 3.8 million adults and more than 500,000 teenagers (mostly female) used tanning booths or sunlamps to tan.

Many users say they get a nice even tan, rather than the red burn they used to get when they tried to cram in too much sun on a short vacation. In a late-1980s study conducted by health educators examining factors that motivated people to use artificial tanning facilities, several common opinions were revealed: tanning is accomplished in less time, a tan is attractive and appealing, the salons have a pleasant atmosphere, and burning is avoided. Many users also believed that tanning beds cure or palliate acne, arthritis, and sinus problems. Others said that they found the salons to be relaxing places where they met friendly people; the ambiance in itself was very appealing. In my own interviews with people who have patronized tanning salons, I noted the same findings but also met a number of people who commented that they wanted to prolong a suntan they had acquired while on vacation; a few admitted that they thought that a tan could camouflage some signs of abusing alcohol or drugs.

Quite a few sun-sensitive people (Type I or II) who otherwise never sunbathe use tanning beds. Why? They know that they have difficulty tanning in the sun, because whenever they try they get a sunburn. But even though they accomplish their goal of tanning without visible burning when they use artificial ultraviolet radiation, they still remain in the category of high risk for skin cancer.

All told, 12 to 24 million people—that is, 5 to 10 percent of the U.S. population—are estimated to use commercial tanning units regularly.

Is UV-A safer than UV-B?

In some ways UV-A is safer, and in other ways it is far more dangerous. You will remember from our discussion in chapter 1 that UV-B can burn the outer layer of the skin more severely but that UV-A penetrates more deeply. These long waves are so intense that about half of them can penetrate to the dermis, which is where the long-term damage occurs. Collagen is lost, your blood vessels decrease in number, and the connective tissue of the dermis is altered. Photoaging is only one hazard, however; skin cancer is a far more serious risk. One reason the tanning bed is appealing is that you probably won't get the blistering kind of sunburn from it that you might get on an island vacation where you are exposed to UV-B as well as UV-A. With artificial tanning, your melanin is stimulated by the penetration of UV-A, so you *may* get a beautiful golden tan.

But while the short-term risks of UV-A are less than those of UV-B, the long-range risks are greater. There is usually a twenty-year time lag between exposure to ultraviolet radiation and development of skin cancer—considerably longer than the period since the inception of these devices.

But aren't tanning devices safer than the sun?

The 1989 report of the National Institutes of Health warns, "Some UV-A lamps generate more than five times more UV-A per unit time than solar UV-A radiation reaching the earth's surface at the equator.

At these doses, even pure UV-A is likely to have adverse biological effects."

And even prior to that report, the Food and Drug Administration had agreed with the American Medical Association and the American Academy of Dermatology when they stated that the claim that these UV-A sunlamps are safer than the sun is very misleading.

People who use tanning booths seem convinced that a good "base tan," gradually achieved, will protect them from sunburn. Some specific research findings, rather than the researchers themselves, have supported that impression. Data derived from studies done with hairless mice indicate that mice first exposed to UV-A radiation similar in wavelength to the UV-A emitted by most tanning salon units, and then exposed to the sun (which emits UV-B as well as UV-A), enjoyed significant protection against the development of skin tumors.

So what does this mean? According to Robert S. Stern, MD, dermatologist at Beth Israel Hospital in Boston, in an editorial in the *Journal of the American Medical Association,* entitled "Beauty Today and Youth Tomorrow?" such data suggest that "at least in the hairless mouse, a brief visit to a tanning parlor before exposure to the sun . . . might help reduce the risk of sun-induced nonmelanoma skin cancer." But then he goes on to explain why the experience of mice in a controlled study like this differs from the way humans experience ultraviolet radiation exposure. The mice had never been exposed to UV-B or sunlight before their exposure to UV-A, whereas humans are. Dr. Stern concludes, "For humans, it is most likely that no matter how acquired, an equal tan results in equal damage to the skin." He concedes that intermittent use of tanning salons may carry a very small risk, but as you know if you have ever used a tanning salon, an occasional session does not produce the cosmetic appearance that most users are seeking.

It is also important to understand that radiation effects are cumulative. Having a tan is equivalent to applying a sunscreen with an SPF (sun protecting factor) of 2 to 4; this simply means that it will take two to four times longer to burn than it would without any protection. But many people, especially those with Type I skin, may *never* be able to build up a protective base. And in any case the UVR protection afforded by a tan is minimal. For this reason, Dr. Stern further states, "Therefore, even if it looks good, a UV-A induced tan does not provide substantial protection from sunburn due to subsequent sun exposure, an often-stated goal of tanning salon users."

Claims that tanning can improve a person's mental state, circulation, or anything else are totally unsubstantiated. There is no known health benefit to be derived from a tan or from exposure to artificial UVR.

Are there any immediate risks of exposure to tanning salons?
The Consumer Product Safety Commission estimates that in a single year there were almost 1,800 hospital emergency room visits for treatment of injuries sustained as a result of time spent at tanning parlors. Most of these accidents were to the eyes—particularly to the cornea. Although consumers are told to wear goggles, many do not heed the instruction, and the UV-A can pass right through the eyelid.

Contrary to some common beliefs, a UV-A tan doesn't protect people from a UV-B sunburn outdoors. Instead, it can augment it and cause a worse burn. One physician reported seeing a man with second-degree burns all over his body; the man had visited a tanning salon, and then followed this exposure with outdoor sunbathing.

Some UV-B may be emitted by tanning beds, and this can cause immediate and painful sunburn even if the tanner doesn't go out in the sun later. Photosensitivity following tanning sessions is often more intense than photosensitivity following outdoor sun exposure. For people taking photosensitive medications or suffering from a photosensitive condition such as lupus, the results can be disastrous. An extreme case occurred in 1989, when a forty-five-year-old woman died from complications caused by burns she suffered at a beauty salon tanning booth. The burns covered 70 percent of her body. This woman reportedly had been taking Psoralen, a photosensitive medication that is often prescribed in conjunction with medically directed and supervised sessions under ultraviolet lamps to treat psoriasis and other skin diseases.

How can you tell when you've had enough?
You can't tell; that's one of the problems with tanning salons. Unlike skin exposed to sunshine, skin exposed to indoor ultraviolet radiation remains cool to the touch, and since you probably won't get an immediate red sunburn (which you might get on the beach), you can't rely on that warning signal.

What are the positions of federal agencies on these devices?
The Food and Drug Administration (FDA) and the Federal Trade Commission (FTC) share responsibility for regulating sunlamps and tanning devices.

The FDA requires manufacturers to place a warning label on all such machines. This label warns consumers that eye and skin injuries, allergic reactions, and long-term risks of skin cancer and premature aging of the skin may result from ultraviolet radiation emitted during exposure. The statement also instructs the user to "WEAR PROTECTIVE EYEWEAR: FAILURE TO DO SO MAY RESULT IN SEVERE BURNS OR LONG-TERM INJURY TO THE EYES. Consult physician before using sunlamp if you are using medications or have a history of skin problems or believe yourself especially sensitive to sunlight. If you do not tan in the sun, you are unlikely to tan from the use of this product."

It sounds like fair warning, doesn't it? But in reality, these signs are not always posted where users can see them. If goggles are not provided, if users are unable to control the unit, and if each unit is not equipped with a working timer, the FDA can recommend that the units be seized—as indeed the U.S. district attorney's office in various jurisdictions can do and often has done. When the problems are corrected, the units may be returned under FDA supervision. As of early 1990, the FDA has not yet called for a total ban on sale of the tanning devices or sunlamps, although many dermatologists are urging that it do so.

The FTC, on the other hand, assumes responsibility for investigating false, misleading, and deceptive advertising claims. If, along with the FDA, the FTC determines that labels or advertisements are not based on valid scientific facts, it has the authority to take corrective action.

The FTC has on many occasions issued orders prohibiting tanning parlors and other companies that have artificial tanning devices from claiming that they do not pose a risk of skin damage to the user. What kind of misleading claims are you likely to see in an advertisement? The FTC distributes a fact sheet that warns against some typical false claims: "You can achieve a deep year-round tan with gentle, comfortable, and safe UV-A light"; "No harsh glare, so no goggles or eye shades are necessary"; "Tan year 'round without the harmful side effects often associated with natural sunlight"; and "No danger in exposure or burning."

The FTC has responded to instances in which firms have made such misleading or false claims by ordering the firms to include the following statement in all or certain ads and promotional materials: "NOTICE–Read the mandatory FDA warning label found on every tanning machine for important information on potential eye injury, skin cancer, skin aging and photosensitive reactions." If this statement appears in the ad, the FTC may (under certain circumstances) permit an ad to claim that its tanning equipment is safe, that it is safer than other devices or other methods of tanning, or that it has health benefits.

If I choose to use these devices, how can I minimize the risks?
Dermatologists hope that you won't ever place yourself under one of these artificial ultraviolet radiation lights. If you do, however, you should make every effort to minimize your risks. According to a report by the American Medical Association's Council on Scientific Affairs in the July 21, 1989, issue of its journal, individuals who insist on using tanning equipment should schedule no more than thirty to fifty half-hour sessions per year.

Using an overall sunscreen isn't very sensible under these circumstances, because you will just have to prolong the tanning sessions to achieve the tan you are seeking. However, if there is some part of your body (such as your nose or lips) that you don't want to tan, cover it with a sunscreen that has an SPF of 15 or higher or with a total block such as zinc oxide. Making use of a tightly woven dry fabric covering in addition to a sunscreen will provide still greater protection. In addition, observe the following safety guidelines:

* Be sure that instructions are posted or photocopied and handed to you, and that they specify the recommended exposure limits for your skin type. And abide by these instructions and recommendations.
* Confirm that there is a manually set timer on the tanning device that will either automatically shut off the lights or somehow signal you (loudly, in the event that you fall asleep) at the end of your predetermined exposure time.
* Safety goggles should be provided.
    — The operator should require that you use the goggles. Any operator's laxity on this score should be taken as a warning signal that the business may not be observing other safety measures.
    — The goggles should fit snugly and should not be cracked. Sunglasses or cotton wads are not acceptable substitutes.
    — The goggles should be sterilized between uses to prevent the spread of any eye infections.
* Check with your physician to ensure that neither the treatment for any condition from which you suffer nor the disease itself is likely to be provoked or exacerbated by ultraviolet radiation.
* Consider any medications you may be taking; antihistamines,

tranquilizers, birth-control pills, and antihypertensives can cause photosensitivity. (See the complete list in appendix II.)

* If you have ever suffered from photosensitivity in the sun, whether as a consequence of chemicals or of allergies, discuss this with your physician. Artificial ultraviolet radiation may trigger the reaction again, this time faster and more intensely. Sunscreens cannot be relied upon to prevent allergic-type reactions in people who are photosensitive.

Operators of tanning salons do not need to obtain an operating license beforehand, and they may be totally ignorant of the risks. In compliance with the FDA, they may hang up the warning sign, without recognizing the long-range or immediate dangers of UVR. Be sure that a qualified attendant is there, or bring a friend with you who can help in an emergency.

According to Dr. Robert S. Stern, in his previously mentioned editorial in the *Journal of the American Medical Association*, "The standards for electrical safety and ultraviolet output of light sources are not stringently regulated in tanning salons." He also lists some of the problems that can arise from poor sanitation in the tanning parlor environment, which can result in a person's acquiring infectious diseases while lying disrobed on the tanning bed. Head lice and skin diseases such as impetigo can be acquired there.

What are the warning signs of injuries, and what should I do about them?
If you have a severe skin burn, an eye burn, or any kind of allergic reaction, seek professional medical attention immediately. Report a new lesion or any change in an existing lesion, mole, or sore to a physician.

If you have followed instructions and still have incurred a serious injury, it is possible that the device may be malfunctioning. Report it to the manufacturer of the device and to the FDA through your local FDA office. Look in the phone book under "U.S. Government, Health and Human Services, Food and Drug Administration."

Tanning Pills

Some tanning pills are promoted as a safe means of tanning; others are meant to bolster resistance to sun damage. Neither should be taken without close medical supervision.

The FDA does not approve of pills that contain beta-carotene and/
or canthaxanthin (although beta-carotene is available by prescription),
both of which are chemical relatives of vitamin A. Sometimes called
French bronzing pills, they are available outside the United States and
occasionally by mail order or through health food stores here. Advertisements sometimes promise "a handsome natural-looking tan without the sun."

According to both the FDA and the Skin Cancer Foundation, some
of the ingredients in these pills have been found to have toxic side
effects. Beta-carotene is a natural component of a number of fruits
and vegetables, including oranges, carrots, and tomatoes. It is sometimes used as a food additive in butter and cheese to add color and in
chicken feed to make egg yolks a brighter yellow. The pills may do
the same thing to you: instead of giving you the handsome melanin-
colored tan you are seeking, they are likely to turn your skin a
jaundicelike yellow or orange.

How does this occur? In combination with the canthaxanthin, beta-
carotene accumulates in the skin, thereby coloring it; but at the same
time it forms deposits in the blood, in fatty tissue, in the liver, and in
other organs, sometimes causing toxicity.

Another kind of pill contains a form of Psoralen, which is used to
treat psoriasis and alopecia areata. Physicians have sometimes prescribed this particular chemical, called 8-methoxypsoralen, for some
people with Type I skin to help increase their resistance to sun
damage. It is theorized that the chemical may thicken the skin and
accelerate melanin production, thus affording the user greater safety
in the sun. It has been recommended by some physicians for certain
individuals who are allergic to sunscreens and cannot avoid the sun.
However, it should only be used under scrupulous medical supervision. Perhaps in the future this treatment will prove to be a satisfactory
way to be safe in the sun, with a suntan. But in the meantime, unless
an experienced dermatologist suggests it, trust the FDA and stay away
from these pills.

Tanning Accelerators

You don't swallow these "guarantees" of a safe tan, at least not literally.
But if you swallow the advertising claims made about tanning accelerators and don't take proper precautions, you will be encouraging
the same sun damage that you would get if you went out in the sun
to burn rather than to tan.

Introduced by a number of major cosmetic companies in the mid-1980s, they continue to be touted as promoters of a fast and deep tan if used once daily for at least three days before sun exposure. The chief ingredient in these products is tyrosine, an amino acid that plays a role in the production of melanin.

Studies done at the prestigious Cleveland Clinic and by *Consumer Reports* magazine of two of these products indicated that the accelerators didn't encourage tanning, with or without sunlight. Reliable and responsible cosmetic and drug companies are continuing to test the products, and they dispute these earlier findings. While the accelerators don't work for everyone, they acknowledge, they purportedly are successful for others. On another front, the FDA is considering whether the claims made for these products are such as to remove them from the category of cosmetics and place them in the category of drugs.

If you do decide to use one of these accelerators (most of the dermatologists I consulted take a wait-and-see attitude toward them), be sure to use a sunscreen, too. Look carefully at labels: some accelerators may combine both in one product. But you need to check the SPF factor in the sunscreen and determine whether it needs to be reapplied regularly.

Sun-free Self-tanners

So-called *bronzers* have been around for many years, and earlier generations of them worked fairly well on men's skin, if carefully applied. But skin with uneven pigmentation or blemishes didn't take kindly to these bronzers, and it was difficult to get them on smoothly, so they didn't work for everyone.

Newer products are far more effective. They look natural, are relatively easy to apply, and are formulated for both men's and women's skin. Some of these products are actually self-tanners that are applied to the skin to give it the color and glow of a tan. These products contain dihydroxyacetone (DHA), an ingredient that safely oxidizes on the skin's surface upon reacting with the protein in the upper layers of the epidermis. In just a few hours, the DHA produces a natural-looking tan that lasts at least three days and won't wash or rub off. As the skin cells renew themselves, the tan fades. Some products of this type incorporate a sunscreen in their formula, but whether they do or not you should be aware that this artificial tan in itself does not give you any more protection from the sun than you would have had without it. If you plan to rely on the built-in sunscreen protection, check to see whether the protection is designed to last as long as the tan. In all likelihood, additional sunscreen must be applied regularly.

Self-tanning products are harmless, but they must be applied with care. They tend to yield less than desirable results for people with uneven skin conditions or facial hair. Keep it away from your hairline, eyebrows, and eyelashes, lest your hair become discolored. It can stain clothing, too, so you must wait for it to dry (about a half-hour) before allowing clothes to come into contact with any part of the skin to which you have applied the product. Wait at least an hour before you shave, bathe, or swim, because these activities can stop the color-developing process.

Transparent gels that you apply to the skin to simulate a tan work in much the same way as the old bronzers, but they have been greatly improved. They are easier to apply, are formulated for men and women, and look very natural. If your skin has many irregularities or you don't want to wait a few hours or you wish to be able to wash the tan away rather than waiting for it to fade, you will like these gels. Other bronzers are brushed in the same manner as blush is and can also give the appearance of a suntan.

According to dermatologists, these products are safe (unless you happen to be allergic to one or more of the ingredients) and offer a healthful alternative to soaking up the sun to achieve a tan.

Summary

Tanning devices, even when they only emit UV-A, are not safe, notwithstanding some advertising claims to the contrary. In fact, they are no safer than the sun and they pose a number of immediate and long-range risks to both skin and eyes. People who choose to use them anyway should observe a number of precautions to minimize risks, particularly to the eyes.

Tanning pills, which typically do not produce a natural-looking tan anyway, have been demonstrated to pose health risks. Tanning accelerators seem safe, but critics and promoters disagree about how effective they are in producing a tan. It is clear, however, that a tan achieved in this way does not provide any screening protection against long-term damage from ultraviolet radiation.

Self-tanners and bronzers, which are topical cosmetic products, are safe alternatives to UV exposure for those who desire a natural-looking tanned appearance. Like tanning accelerators, these products do not produce a UVR-blocking tan.

4 *Black Skin*

"You're so lucky that you don't have to worry about the sun," Sandra's Caucasian friends tell her.

"Not so," says Sandra, an African-American who is a human resources administrator at a large medical center, "although it's true my skin ages more slowly than white skin does. Some people say that's because black skin has a greater abundance of oil glands and larger pores to keep it well-lubricated; but a number of experts say that the reason black-skinned people have such youthful skin is because of their natural protection from the sun. My risks of cancer are lower than Caucasians', too, but they're not nil. So I use a sunscreen before outdoor events, and last year we put up a big awning on the deck so we can stay out of the direct sun when we entertain. All our guests—black, white, and Asian—appreciate it."

Ultraviolet Radiation

Sandra knows that the partial destruction of the earth's protective ozone layer means that considerably more ultraviolet radiation, both UV-A and UV-B, is reaching earth. Although, studies indicate the potential for damage to blacks from ultraviolet radiation is far less than that to whites, the threat does exist.

The Skin

In chapter 2 we noted that the skin cells known as *melanocytes* are responsible for producing melanin, which determines the skin's pigmentation and provides some defense against ultraviolet radiation. The number of melanocytes remains the same for all people, but in dark-skinned people the melanocytes are larger, more active, and more widely dispersed.

The structure of the stratum corneum (the outer layer of the epidermis) differs between Caucasians and African-Americans. The thickness of the layer is probably the same for everyone, although there is some dispute about that, but the cell structure of the stratum corneum in blacks is more compact and less porous and has more cell layers than in whites. For this reason, black skin is somewhat more resistant to chemical irritation and constitutes a more effective barrier against penetration from the environment. In a number of studies it has been demonstrated that black skin is far more successful than white skin at barring both UV-A and UV-B. The amount of time a person with dark skin can remain in the sun before getting burned (called the MED or minimal erythema dose) may be as much as thirty-three times that of a fair-skinned person. However, black skin is by no means thirty-three times better than white skin at screening out the sun.

Effects of the Sun

Using a sunscreen is a good practice for everyone to adopt, since a sunburn can be painful. It may be difficult for a black person to tell at once when the skin is getting burned, because it may not become darker right away. But the exposed skin can feel tender, warm, and tight, and it may itch; swelling and blistering may also occur. Sun poisoning can cause nausea, chills, and fever. Mild sunburn usually responds to nonprescription sunburn remedies. Soaking in a cool bath is often helpful at subduing swelling and inflammation and even acting as an anesthetic for the skin. Sunburn on the lips is not uncommon and can be very painful. Therefore, protection for the skin and especially for the lips is essential. If any symptoms of sunburn persist or worsen, see a physician.

Studies have established that melanin cannot be depended upon entirely to protect skin against the sun. Just as a suntan does not offer a Caucasian person complete protection against sunburn, possessing naturally dark skin as a result of a large amount of melanin does not give an African-American such protection. In both cases, it's like sitting under an umbrella in the sun: you have some defense, but not total protection.

Everyone needs vitamin D for strong bones. It prevents rickets in children, and is also important for adults and the elderly. Vitamin D is manufactured in the skin by the ultraviolet component of sunlight, and dark-skinned people are at a disadvantage in producing it because their melanin screens out much of the sun's ultraviolet radiation. Thus, maintaining a diet that includes vitamin-D-fortified foods is quite important. A good supplementary multivitamin will also contain the vitamin D required.

Although cancer of the skin is the most common form of cancer in the general population, it remains relatively rare among African-

Americans. However, various studies indicate that those who do develop skin cancer tend to get it in the sun-exposed areas of their body. So although your skin cancer risks diminish, the darker-skinned you are, hazards still exist.

At the annual meeting of the American Academy of Dermatology in December 1989, George T. Reizner, MD, of the University of Wisconsin-Madison Medical School told his colleagues that—although light-skinned Caucasians continue to have the greatest rate of skin cancer—the rate is increasing for African-Americans, Hispanics, and Asian-Americans. He noted that the increase is concentrated in cancers related to exposure to the sun and its ultraviolet rays. This demonstrates the need for everyone, regardless of skin color, to take precautions when they participate in outdoor activities, either for pleasure or for work.

In addition, any of the problems that strike light-skinned people who bask in the sun can also attack dark-skinned people. For instance, there is evidence that sun exposure can weaken your immune system, leaving you vulnerable to diseases from the common cold to cancer. People who suffer from systemic lupus erythematosus (and they include many blacks, women in particular)—a chronic, inflammatory disease that affects many systems of the body—are often extremely sensitive to the sun. Indeed, exposure can trigger a life-threatening flare-up in some individuals.

Although clear differences exist between black and white skins, it is virtually impossible to make accurate generalizations about the characteristics of black skin, according to Harold E. Pierce, MD, assistant professor of dermatology at the Howard University College of Medicine in Washington, D.C. Most African-Americans reflect a blend of African, European, and American Indian forebears, and the pigmentation of black skin may range from very light to very dark.

Problems That Beset Black Skin

Some skin problems of African-Americans are not as likely to occur among white-skinned people. For instance, differences in the structure of connective tissue make black skin more vulnerable to scarring, scaling, and forming small pimplelike lesions in reaction to cuts and scrapes, and may give rise to *keloids*—elevated fibrous tissue that is hard, shiny, smooth, thick, dark, and rubbery.

All skin has some response to trauma, ranging from a minor scratch to pimples, acne, eczema, allergies, psoriasis (less common among African-Americans than among Caucasians), and any kind of inflammation. Black skin often responds to trauma by producing either hyperpigmentation (increased pigmentation) or hypopigmentation (loss of pigmentation); what determines whether the body will respond with hypo- or hyperpigmentation is not known.

These conditions are difficult and time-consuming to treat, and treatment is not always successful. Sometimes the problem clears up by itself over a period of time, so most dermatologists recommend using a cosmetic cover-up while waiting for normal pigmentation to return.

Between 2 and 5 percent of African-Americans experience a disorder called *vitiligo*, in which areas of the skin lack pigmentation. This is a progressive condition that can be deeply upsetting emotionally to the sufferer. Vitiligo is not hazardous to the health, unless (as in rare instances) it is associated with other medical problems such as pernicious anemia, some disease of the thyroid or adrenal gland, or secondary syphilis. The loss of pigmentation occurs when the melanocytes in an area of skin shut down operation and no melanin is produced. Vitiligo is thought to be a type of autoimmune condition in which the body rejects some of its own cells. It can affect one part of the body, a few small areas, or extensive regions. Frequently it appears on the backs of the hands, on the face (especially around the mouth and eyes), and on the genitals. It may occur symmetrically, or not.

Vitiligo is often treated with PUVA (also used for stubborn cases of psoriasis), making use of Psoralen alone or in combination with other drugs. Psoralen is a light-sensitizing medication that is applied topically to the skin or taken orally prior to ultraviolet light treatment. This therapy is provided in a doctor's office, usually by a dermatologist; it is not something you can do on your own. Hundreds of treatments may be necessary, and even then it is not always cosmetically successful. During the treatment period, normal skin will also darken, making the vitiligo appear more obvious than usual. Applying a sunscreen to the area may help mitigate this effect. Patients have to wear UV-A-screening sunglasses or goggles during treatments.

According to some studies, less than 70 percent of people with vitiligo have a favorable response to the PUVA treatment; consequently some physicians suggest that patients with extensive vitiligo consider achieving a more evenly pigmented appearance by applying bleach to the unaffected skin. This procedure, too, *must* be done under medical supervision. However, bleaching means that the individual will end up with very light (perhaps white) skin, and this may not be cosmetically or emotionally satisfactory. Some additional treatments for repigmenting affected areas are being tested, and others are on the horizon, but many men and women just choose to live with vitiligo, using one of the various commercially available concealers and cover-up cosmetics that can be blended into the surrounding pigmented skin very effectively.

The absence of melanin in areas affected by vitiligo can leave these areas totally unprotected and highly susceptible to damage from the sun. For this reason, anyone who has vitiligo or hypopigmentary areas must take considerable precautions before venturing into the sun.

Albinism, an inborn condition characterized by partial or total absence of pigmentation, occurs in all races of humans. The skin and eyes of albinos are supersensitive to the sun and must be protected from it completely. In addition to serious eye problems, those who were exposed to considerable UVR often developed basal cell cancers and melanomas; and died very young.

African and East Asian skin, more than European skin, has a tendency to form keloid scars that are large, permanent, and sometimes deforming. They may occur after surgery or following any injury to the skin, including severe, blistering sunburn. Although keloids can appear anywhere on the body, they develop most frequently in the area between the breasts, on the upper chest, and in the area between the shoulder blades. The scar may extend even beyond the trauma site. Treatment of keloids is difficult because of their tendency to recur and enlarge if they are surgically removed. Sometimes corticosteroid injections are used to shrink them; often the keloids are first frozen with liquid nitrogen to soften them; sometimes steroids are used in combination with surgery. Such treatments should only be undertaken by an experienced and knowledgeable physician.

Hypertrophic scars, often referred to as *proud flesh,* is another condition in which excessive tissue, in the form of scars, rises above the skin. In appearance, they can be purplish red and are firm and rubbery. Although hypertrophic scars do not usually grow very large, they can cause itching and discomfort. They sometimes disappear on their own over a period of time, but if this doesn't occur they are usually treated with injections of corticosteroids. Hypertrophic scars are not generally thought of as being closely tied to sun exposure, but it is wise to remember that anything that causes injury or scarring of the skin can lead to this condition.

Actinic keratoses (sun-induced precancerous lesions) and squamous cell cancers may develop in the sites of long-standing discoid lupus (a chronic, recurrent disease that primarily affects the skin). Certain chemicals and medications you may come into contact with can cause photosensitivity, an adverse skin reaction resulting from combined exposure to ultraviolet radiation and a particular chemical substance. The natural resistance to sun damage many African-Americans enjoy is no guarantee of protection against adverse reaction resulting from photosensitivity.

African-Americans are as likely as Caucasions to suffer from one of the *porphyrias*—a general term for a group of inherited disorders in which the body abnormally constructs certain parts of hemoglobin molecules in red blood cells. These substances then act as photosensitizers and can cause erosions, scars, and severe hyperpigmentation.

Because early cancerous lesions may not be as readily apparent on dark skin as they are on lighter skin, it is especially important for dark-skinned people to practice the early detection methods outlined in chapters 7 and 8 on cancers. Malignant melanoma, a serious and life-threatening skin cancer, is rarer in blacks than in whites, but it can easily be overlooked or unrecognized and thus remain undiagnosed and untreated in its early stages when it is still highly curable.

Dark eye color does not offer protection against the effects of ultraviolet radiation on eyes, so African-Americans should be sure to wear sunglasses (either prescription or nonprescription) that block out ultraviolet radiation. This subject is discussed fully in chapter 6.

Sandra, whom you met a few pages earlier, synopsized the relationship between black skin and the sun as follows: "I might not have to worry as much about the sun causing cancer or premature skin aging, but if I were to have a bad sunburn or a severe reaction to the sun, it might leave me with keloids or unattractive pigmentation disorders. So believe me, I'm not looking for any unnecessary problems. I'm very careful about the sun: I never go out without a sunscreen. My husband and I always use it, even sitting on our deck under the awning in midsummer. And we wear sunglasses that screen out UVR."

Summary

Black skin differs from white skin in its amount of pigmentation—the result of larger, more widely dispersed, and more active melanocytes.

The melanin produced by these cells offers the body protection against damage from ultraviolet radiation.

Although dark-skinned people have far lower rates of skin cancer than do light-skinned people, they are not immune to it. Various other skin problems affect African-Americans, and some of these may be caused or exacerbated by exposure to the sun. Photosensitivity can occur in people of all races, and black skin often responds to trauma (including sunburn) with hyperpigmentation or hypopigmentation, either of which is extremely difficult to treat medically. However, excellent cosmetic products are available for concealing uneven skin color.

African-Americans should be careful to protect themselves from the sun, either by wearing protective clothing or by using a sunscreen on exposed parts of their body and face. Individuals who have areas of hypopigmentation must take special precautions to avoid sun exposure. And finally, wear sunglasses that screen out ultraviolet radiation.

5

The Youngest Skin: Infants, Children, and Adolescents

There was a time when parents believed that if their child didn't get plenty of sunshine and have the suntan to prove it, the youngster was being deprived of some of the best things in life.

We know better now, but old habits are hard to break, and at any family pool party or backyard barbecue you can hear fond relatives admiringly say, "He looks terrific; he has such a nice tan." And the lucky family who returns from Disneyworld in midwinter, or a week with Grandma in Arizona may be greeted by children and adults alike who say, "You must have had wonderful weather; you have such a healthy tan."

But the reality is that no tan is healthy. Still, most people love the way they look with a tan, and according to Sidney Hurwitz, MD, Clinical Professor of Pediatrics and Dermatology at the Yale University School of Medicine, "Suntanned skin has now become a badge of affluence, sex appeal, health, and personal self-esteem. Thus, young children and teenagers, as well as adults, have become preoccupied with suntanning."

Melanin is produced as the skin's response to injury; adding pigment to the skin serves as a natural means of attempting to protect it. But damage does occur, and by the time people are in their twenties, those who were exposed to the sun early in life are actually showing subtle signs of aging. Each year of sun exposure contributes to earlier wrinkling, blotching, and drying of skin, and to the earlier onset of precancerous lesions and cancer itself. Statistics indicate that this is happening to younger and younger people.

According to a May 1989 report by the National Institutes of Health, data suggest that 50 percent of an individual's total lifetime ultraviolet radiation exposure occurs by the age of eighteen. A number of experts have estimated that, by the age of twenty, a person has received 70 to 80 percent of his or her lifetime of UVR exposure. Dr. Hurwitz reminds us that children have many more opportunities to be exposed to midday sun than do adults. "It is estimated," he says, "that the average child receives three times more annual UVB than the average adult."

No wonder. How many adults get a few months off each summer to explore in the park, play in the backyard, frolic in the pool, ocean, or lake, and ride their bikes on the sidewalk? Thus, children need sensible protection from the sun from the time they are born. Their tender skin soaks up the sun, and although they may not develop an acute sunburn they are setting the stage later for skin cancer. In its public awareness campaigns, the Skin Cancer Foundation states, "It takes years to get skin cancer and most of us get an early start." Even though most people know that the sun causes skin cancer (in fact, the sun is responsible for at least 90 percent of all skin cancers) and premature aging, many of them are unaware of the increasing evidence that continuous sun exposure during childhood is a major risk factor in developing skin cancers in adulthood. According to current studies, regular use of sunscreen with an SPF of 15 during the first eighteen years of life would reduce a person's lifetime risk of developing nonmelanoma skin cancer by 78 percent. Melanoma, a far more serious and life-threatening skin cancer, has been associated with brief but intense exposures and blistering sunburns in childhood.

A study done in Greensland, Australia, makes this clear. Australia has the highest rate of malignant melanoma in the world: it is ten times higher than the rate in the British Isles, where sunlight exposure is far less, but where people have similar heredity and skin types. Several years ago, scientists in Australia decided to address this problem by conducting careful research. They learned that a person's teenage and young adult years were a critical time for the deleterious effects of sun exposure to occur and that, from the point of view of melanoma risk, ages ten to twenty-four are the worst time of life to live in a sunny climate.

Harvard Medical School dermatologist Arthur J. Sober, MD, and other researchers have demonstrated that individuals who experience even one blistering sunburn in adolescence double their risk of developing melanoma later. At the National Institutes of Health conference in 1989, Dr. Sober referred to studies from Israel and New Zealand, as well as from Australia, demonstrating that fair-skinned people who were born in these countries or who migrated there early in life had higher rates of melanoma than those who arrived later in childhood. Obviously, the earlier and longer you reside in an environment characterized by hot sun, the greater your opportunity for experiencing an early intense sunburn will be. A number of studies indicate that the development of other skin cancers results from suntanning over a more extended period of time.

This information should make it clear that—whether you live in the sunbelt, where exposure is fairly steady and cumulative, or in a temperate climate but have occasional vacations in the sun—children need a lifetime of protection to avoid skin cancer. How do we protect babies', children's, and adolescents' skin? Not by denying them the pleasures of summer fun or winter vacations in warm climates, but by beginning sun safety habits when they are youngsters. Just as you allow your children to have occasional sweets but make certain that they brush their teeth regularly, and an additional time after sticky sweets, so you can let them enjoy the sunshine if they routinely use a sunscreen and take extra precautions when exposure is especially potent. Whenever possible, they should stay out of the sun between 10 A.M. and 3 P.M. These habits will continue to pay dividends if they carry over into adulthood.

Young Babies

Look in a newborn nursery or peer into carriages, and you will notice that most babies have fair skin and blue or light eyes. That's because their pigment protection is not complete at birth. Even children who will later have brown eyes and dark, deeply pigmented skin are fairly light at birth. Slowly the skin color changes and begins to correspond more closely to that of the parents. There is a relationship between the state of the pigment system and eye color: as long as eyes remain blue (and some people will always have blue eyes), the pigment system is light, and such an individual remains at high risk for sun damage.

Babies do not need to spend substantial time in the sun. If Grandma says they do in order to get their vitamin D, assure her that just the bit of sunlight your baby gets while accompanying you in the carriage on a walk to a neighbor's house or to do a few errands will provide plenty of vitamin D. Moreover, breast-fed babies of well-nourished mothers, as well as bottle-fed babies on formula or vitamin-D-fortified milk, get enough vitamin D to provide their bones with what they need without any sunshine, although many pediatricians recommend a vitamin supplement that includes vitamin D.

The sunscreen companies themselves and a number of physicians do not recommend sunscreens for babies under the age of six months. Ask your pediatrician before deciding whether or not to use sunscreen. But if the answer is, "Wait six months," the only effective protection you can provide is to restrict sun exposure during that time. And such protection should begin on the trip home from the hospital. Later, if the family wants to go to the beach for the day, be sure that you bring a tightly woven umbrella and that the baby is also wearing a lightweight but tightly woven hat. Try to limit your excursions during this critical period to short stays, go where you know you can find plenty of shade, and be sure that the carriage or blanket is well shielded from the sun. A carriage with a hood will shield your baby's face better than an upright stroller will. If you do use a stroller, attach a canopy or an umbrella to it. Sand, concrete, snow, and water can reflect ultraviolet radiation, so if you have a choice, place the carriage on grass rather than on a patio, and if you're at the beach, stay away from the water, and spread an old blanket or bedspread under the carriage. Don't relax your vigilance on overcast days, because 80 percent of the sun's radiation can penetrate the clouds.

The skin constitutes a larger percentage of the total body mass of babies than of adults, so they are especially vulnerable to anything that affects their skin. For instance, says Henry E. Wiley, III, MD, Assistant Clinical Professor of Pediatrics at the University of Florida, Gainsville, and a member of the Medical Council of the Skin Cancer Foundation, "A bad sunburn in an infant might cause serious fluid and electrolyte problems. The same burn in an adult might be intensely painful but not an immediate threat."

What about Grandma's advice to place the baby in a carriage near a sunny window? Most closed windows effectively screen out UV-B, but they may only screen out some of the UV-A. So if you do this, be sure to shield the baby's skin and eyes from ultraviolet radiation.

Whenever possible, avoid taking babies outdoors at midday on hot, sunny days. If you are about to go stir-crazy, or if you have other demands that require you to leave the house and you don't have a sitter, then by all means go out, but take time to ensure that the baby is well protected from the sun.

Older Babies, Toddlers, and Children

After a baby reaches the age of six months, there is no controversy about using a sunscreen, and many manufacturers make them especially for children. Most do not contain PABA, a common sunscreen ingredient that can be irritating to children's (and many adults') skin. Unscented screens are good because they are less likely to attract insects. Buy one with an SPF (sun protection factor) of at least 15, manufactured by a major drug company that you trust; and buy it at a store that has a big turnover, so you can be confident that it hasn't already been around for a few seasons. Look for the expiration date on the box; if there isn't one, the sunscreen probably doesn't contain ingredients that lose their potency over time. Even though a sunscreen has been shown to be safe and effective, it is a good idea to test it on your child several days before you plan to rely on it for extended periods of protection, to be sure it won't cause photosensitivity or allergies. Dr. Wiley suggests that you apply a small amount to an area removed from the face (such as the arm or abdomen); if redness or irritation appear in the area of the application, select another product. He says that, in general, creamy sunscreens work better for young children because they are less drying to skin, can be seen more easily during application, and stay on longer. They are also less likely than lotions to contain alcohol, which might sting. Apply the sunscreen carefully to the face, circling around the eyes but avoiding the upper and lower eyelids. Sunscreens also come in stick form, which is useful for lips, scalp, nose, and ears. The sunscreen should be applied liberally (don't stint on it!) on all uncovered areas and under sheer clothing. You can't expect a thin T-shirt or lacy bathing suit to offer full protection from the sun's rays—especially if it gets wet—so be particularly diligent about applying sunscreen under lightweight clothes. Sunscreen should be applied fifteen or thirty minutes before exposure, because it takes time for all the active ingredients to sink into the skin. In Part Two we will discuss sunscreens in more detail. (See appendix 1 for information about sunscreens that have received the Seal of Recommendation by the Skin Cancer Foundation.)

Dr. Wiley says that zinc oxide (that old standard used by lifeguards and golfers) has a long safety record in the very young; it can be used in addition to a sunscreen and on vulnerable places such as the nose, the cheeks, the tops of the ears, and the shoulders.

A child in a stroller or sandbox should be wearing a sunscreen during warm-weather days, whether or not the sun is visibly strong. Waterproof sunscreens are best, even when a dip in the pool, lake, or ocean isn't on the agenda, because children play with water toys, need frequent face washing, and may go running through the sprinkler in the backyard or playground.

Protection from the sun is vital for all children, but according to the Skin Cancer Foundation's pamphlet "For Every Child Under the Sun," special care must be taken if a child has one or more of the following risk factors:

Fair skin and/or freckles
Blonde, red, or light brown hair
Blue, green, or gray eyes
A tendency to burn easily and to tan little or not at all
A tendency to burn before tanning
A family history of skin cancer
Residence in a warm, sunny climate
Long periods of daily exposure or short periods of intense exposure
A large number of moles

In chapter 2 we discussed photosensitivity—an adverse response to sunlight, resulting in a rash, redness, and/or swelling, following exposure to both the sun and certain medications. If a child has been taking an antibiotic or any other medication, discuss this with the physician or pharmacist before letting the child spend much time in the sun. Sunscreens that guard against UV-A as well as UV-B offer some (but not always adequate) protection against photosensitivity.

If your child is born with large moles, called *congenital nevi,* or acquires them shortly after birth, be sure that the pediatrician takes a good look at them; it may also be wise to take the child to a dermatologist. In addition to congenital nevi, unusual moles known as *dysplastic nevi* (which usually don't appear before adolescence) signal a slightly increased risk of developing malignant melanoma later. They too should be carefully examined by a physician. The Skin Cancer Foundation recommends that you inspect your child's skin regularly (after a bath is a good time), watching for any new raised growths, itchy patches, nonhealing sores, changes in moles, or new colored areas. Although skin cancer is extremely rare in children and uncommon in teenagers, it is never too soon to establish a regimen for caring for the health of the skin.

Most of us tend to think of hot weather as the time to be most careful about the sun, but remember that snow reflects the sun even more effectively than sand or water does. So while sledding or skiing, children can get a heavy dose of ultraviolet radiation. In addition, anytime you are at a high altitude—such as on the ski slopes—the amount of ambient UVR increases.

Be sure that your children take precautions whenever they engage in outdoor activities. Find out whether your children's schools, camps, athletic programs, day-care centers, and other institutions schedule such activities at the safest times, and whether the teachers and counselors apply sunscreen to younger children, remind the older ones to use it, or even provide it for those who might have forgotten to bring it with them.

If your children regularly swim at an outdoor pool, you may be interested to know that some communities and private clubs do not permit swimmers to wear T-shirts, because fibers can clog the pool's filter system. Many pools have ordinances requiring a shower before swimming. This can wash away a sunscreen, which is probably at least part of the intention, since the oils from sunscreens can cling to the pool's tile. Try to lobby against this, because ultraviolet radiation reaches you in the water and is reflected back at you from the bottom of the pool. Apply a good waterproof sunscreen if the youngster is to spend more than a few minutes in the water, and instruct him or her to take the mandatory preswim shower without soap.

Insist that your children wear sunglasses on sunny days, and make sure they have sunglasses on when they ski or sled for long periods of time. These help to protect sensitive young eyes and eyelids, preventing cumulative damage that might otherwise lead to cataract formation in later years. For more on eye care, see chapter 6.

Adolescents

Try to tell the teenagers in your family something, and in all likelihood they will nod intelligently and do what they want, listen respectfully and promptly forget it, or not even appear to have heard one word you said. Therefore, I can't guarantee that they will listen to me; but it's definitely worth a try. And it's important that *you* know what can be done about protecting your teenager from the effects of UVR.

When you're young, it's difficult to believe that anything you are doing now will seriously affect your life later. Sure, you might believe that studying for exams will help you get into college, which will then help you get a better job—but that's only a few years down the line. Nineteen-year-old college students aren't likely to worry that in twenty years they will be faced with the need to pay for tuition for their children. When you remind a pair of sixteen-year-olds that all those french fries and hamburgers are going to raise their cholesterol level and increase their risk of having a heart attack when they turn forty-six, they usually aren't very impressed—at least not enough to do something about it. So you can see how difficult it can be to impress upon them the importance of being careful in the sun and of not getting a tan because it will lead to premature aging and cancer—even if you use language as catchy as the American Cancer Society slogan, "Fry now, pay later."

A teenager who read the first few chapters of this book would have a clear picture of the effects of the sun on skin. It's almost certain that a steady diet of sun will lead to some wrinkles before thirty, lots of them by forty, and precancerous lesions before fifty. It can also lead to a far more serious form of skin cancer, malignant melanoma. Arthur J. Sober, MD, states, "By midteens, appreciable numbers of melanomas are seen. In New Zealand, for example, one-third of melanomas occur in the under-40 age group."

Many adolescents know that sun exposure can lead to this result (although most are surprised to learn it can happen so soon), but they love the way they look with a tan, and they eagerly embrace the mistaken idea that artificial sources of UVR are safe. According to a National Institutes of Health panel, adolescents and young adults form the largest category of the 1 million Americans who make use of commercial tanning facilities every day. See chapter 3 for a discussion of why many dermatologists believe that tanning salons should be banned.

Neither the sun nor artificial UVR can cure acne, although many young people afflicted with it believe that it will. Acne sometimes does improve in the summer, and it is possible that the sun has a somewhat ameliorative effect on some people's skin, but a dermatologist can advise much safer and more effective ways than exposure to the sun to clear it up.

Adolescents often assert that before long they will be "chained" to a desk in an office, and so they argue that these summers are their last chance to enjoy the outdoors. A part-time or full-time job that entails considerable outdoor activity, such as mowing lawns, working at a beach or pool club, parking cars, or baby-sitting, may offer as one of its main attractions the opportunity to "work on a tan." Deciding to forgo a tan and be safe in the sun may not be easy for teens to do. But if they could meet some of the young people who have shared their stories through the Skin Cancer Foundation, they might reconsider going unprotected into the beautiful glowing sun.

A pretty, vivacious sixteen-year-old named Sandy tells about spending a lot of time at the beach at Cape Cod. Sandy isn't a sun-worshiper; she simply enjoyed water activities and became an enthusiastic waterskier. On a few occasions, she got badly sunburned and began to peel. Afterward, at her mother's urging, she stayed out of the sun for a few days. But when school began in the fall, she noticed a sore on the side of her nose where she had been sunburned, and it just didn't go away; instead, it grew larger, became crusty, and began oozing. She went to a dermatologist, who did a biopsy with a long needle, removing a piece of tissue. The report came back from the lab with a clear diagnosis: basal cell carcinoma. Sandy knew what this was because not too long before she had seen President Reagan on television with a bandage on his nose, describing his skin cancer. "Kids don't get skin cancer," she had thought, until it happened to her.

Over and over, stories like Sandy's are repeated in dermatologists' offices. Although basal cell skin cancers are curable, you can look quite unattractive during the time before treatment is completed and healing has taken place. Sandy's treatment involved four different surgical procedures to ensure that all the cancer cells had been removed and that a layer of healthy cells now surrounded the place where the cancerous sore had once been. (This is called *Mohs surgery* and will be discussed in full in Part Three.) Sometimes a person is left with a large, disfiguring hole where the cancer was removed, requiring plastic surgery to restore a normal appearance.

Malignant melanoma frequently strikes people in the twenty-to-forty age group. This is a life-threatening disease that often begins with a mole that either suddenly appears or changes in size, shape, or color. Malignant melanoma is discussed in chapter 8, but it is important to note here that the teenage years are a key time when sun exposure—especially one or more severe cases of sunburn—sets the stage for development of this disease. Although melanoma is curable when recognized early, the life of a person who has had it may be forever changed. Many dermatologists and other physicians recommend that a young woman who has had melanoma not plan on becoming pregnant for many years—or perhaps ever—because pregnancy can activate hormones that are implicated in the onset of melanoma. And anyone who has had melanoma must be exceedingly careful to stay out of the sun thenceforth; the disease can recur even after it has been diagnosed at an early stage and seemingly cured.

Does this mean that to be safe you and your children have to give up sailing, waterskiing, swimming, vacations in the sun, or jobs that keep you outdoors? Not at all: the conscientious use of sunscreens, UV-blocking sunglasses, and clothes that help shield you from the sun will give you the protection and assurance you need. Part Two of this book describes the steps involved in protecting yourself from the sun and from ultraviolet radiation.

It's easy to remind yourself and your children to wear sunscreen when packing your picnic, bathing suit, and towel to go off to the countryside or to the beach. But Dr. Wiley notes that parents sometimes forget about sun exposure when it is linked to a practical activity such as mowing the lawn, walking the dog, or washing the car. Keep in mind that sun is sun; and protection should be in place before you or your children embark on any activities that occur under its rays. It is wiser to schedule these outdoor chores before 10 A.M. or after 3 P.M., especially in summer or in the Sun Belt. Store sunscreens in convenient, readily accessible areas where they are likely to be used.

Ultraviolet Radiation as Therapy

In chapter 2 we discussed the use of ultraviolet light in conjunction with particular medications to treat skin disorders such as psoriasis, vitiligo, and alopecia areata. Such treatments may be beneficial to children who suffer from these conditions, but they should *never* be attempted by a parent alone; instead, they should only be administered under careful medical supervision. Even under these conditions, however, UV treatments may place a youngster at a higher risk for skin cancer later. Therefore, if possible, other treatments should be attempted before a method that uses ultraviolet light is employed.

Parental Initiative in Being Safe in the Sun

A 1986 study found that, although 90 percent of the mothers interviewed associated skin cancer with overexposure to sunlight, only half of them faithfully applied sunscreen to their children's skin. Increasingly, though, parents are recognizing the importance of protecting their children from ultraviolet radiation; so as more effective and easier-to-apply sunscreens become available, this number should increase. Take the trouble to be among the group of parents who make certain that their children are protected from the sun. It is a significant investment in their future health.

Summary

Although a child with a suntan may look healthy and glowing, the reality is that exposure to the sun starting in early years simply gives a person a head start on developing skin cancer.

Youngsters need protection from the sun at all ages. Babies younger than six months, because they do not yet have their complete pigment protection, should be completely shielded from sunlight; and after six months, they should be protected with efficient sunscreens. Children who are in the high-risk category because of light coloring, family history of skin cancer, habitation in a warm, sunny climate, frequent sun exposure, or possession of a large number of moles require particularly diligent protection.

It is often difficult to convince adolescents that they need to protect their skin in order to avoid premature aging and cancer later on. Teens need to be aware that, while the incidence is uncommon, they *can* develop skin cancers and melanoma now—not just when they are a lot older. Parents can help their children organize their outdoor schedules at times when sun is less intense and can provide appropriate clothing, sunscreens, and sunglasses.

Parental involvement with schools, camps, and athletic programs in order to obtain cooperation in both outdoor scheduling and the provision of sunscreen is also beneficial.

6 The Sun and the Eyes

Back in the days when I considered a suntan glamorous and thought that it was even healthful to stretch out in the sun, I avoided sunglasses. Wearing them resulted in "panda marks," as we teenagers called those white circles surrounding our eyes where the sunglasses had successfully screened out the sun.

Then when I got a little older I noticed that, if I didn't wear sunglasses for reading outdoors, I would squint and get crinkley little lines all around my eyes—lines that were beginning to look like wrinkles. So on went the sunglasses, at least for reading in the sun.

I learned a few more important lessons when I married a man whose daughter is an ophthalmologist. She's Jacqueline Lustgarten, MD, an associate clinical professor of ophthalmology at the Mount Sinai School of Medicine in New York. As a member of the American Academy of Ophthalmology, she is a medical doctor, educated, trained, and licensed to provide complete medical eye care. She's very strict about matters relating to eyes, both with patients and with her own family. When her father argued that he didn't think he needed glasses for driving, she said, "Well, if you plan on driving my children, you'd better wear them." And when her family skis, her sons don't dare go up on the slopes without sunscreen and sunglasses.

Structures and Function of Eyes

Sight is one of our most important senses; many people feel that it is the one they would most regret losing. And yet many of us don't take proper care of our eyes, perhaps because we don't really understand their structure or how they work.

Eyes need light in order to fulfill their function as the sensory organ of vision. Many of us see better in daylight than in artificial light, but ironically the visible portion of ultraviolet radiation also represents a threat to the well-being of the tissues of the eye.

Our eyes work harder than most of us realize. Like a camera, the eye also has a lens through which light passes before focusing on the retina, the thin light-sensitive film that lines the inside of the eye. A chemical reaction takes place there in which, as on the film in a camera, an image is briefly recorded.

The region of the eye, or *ocular area,* consists of many parts. Eyebrows help to protect eyes by preventing rain and sweat from running down into them. Eyelids are also protective. They work like shutters, allowing the eyes to rest; and they blink quickly (this is called the *blink reflex*) if anything comes too close. Glands in the eyelids produce tears, washing the eye every few seconds during the blink reflex. Eyelashes trap dust, dirt, raindrops, and snowflakes that might otherwise fall into the eye.

The structure of the eye itself is complex and intricate. The eyeball (globe) fits into the socket (orbit), a skeletal pocket in the skull. Covering most of the eyeball and the inside of the eyelid is the conjunctiva, a transparent lining. This membrane sometimes gets infected, causing conjunctivitis, which some people refer to as *pink eye*. The conjunctiva manufactures oily secretions that prevent friction from occurring when the eye moves. It can also become red and irritated from allergies.

The eye is composed of elaborate layers, each of which serves a specific purpose. The outer layer consists of the tough but sensitive cornea and sclera. The sclera is the white of the eye, which protects it from injury and irritation. The cornea, an extension of the sclera at the front of the eye, acts as a transparent window through which light can pass. The cornea covers and protects the iris, the colored part of the eye, but is extremely sensitive itself, as you know if you have ever felt a particle of sand or an eyelash scratch against it. The iris expands and contracts to widen or narrow the pupil, the opening at its center, thus controlling the amount of light that passes through to the layers behind it. When too much light is directed toward the eye, the pupil gets smaller, allowing a narrower stream of light in. When there is insufficient light, the pupil opens wide, permitting as much available light as possible to enter.

Behind the pupil is a natural lens that, in a person's normal state, is so clear that light can pass right through it. This flexible structure focuses light by altering its shape. The lens is held in place by muscles and ligaments that help it focus. The lens is flat and thin when you look at things in the distance, but it becomes short and fat when you look at something close to you.

In front of the lens is an area termed the *anterior chamber;* it is filled with a watery fluid that helps maintain the proper pressure inside the eye. Attached to the innermost lining of the eyeball is the retina, which receives the image that the lens has refracted or bent. The retina is made up of many nerve endings that act as light receptors. Cells called *cones* and *rods* (approximately 6 million and 120 million of each, respectively) transmit the images to the optic nerve at the back of the eye. The cones work in bright light and pick up colors; the rods work in dim light and cannot register color but are important for peripheral vision and in seeing light, shape, and movement. The area behind the lens and in front of the retina is filled with a jellylike substance called *vitreous humor,* which is colorless and clear.

When the optic nerve receives the images from the cones and rods, it transmits the messages to the visual centers of the brain. Interestingly, the retina, like a camera, receives these pictures "upside-down," but the brain turns them around.

What Can Go Wrong?

Now that we have seen how the eyes normally work and how the brain receives their messages, let's consider what can go wrong. The eyes don't always work perfectly: some people have minor vision problems that are correctable with eyeglasses, and more serious conditions (such as those described next) may require complex treatment and even surgery.

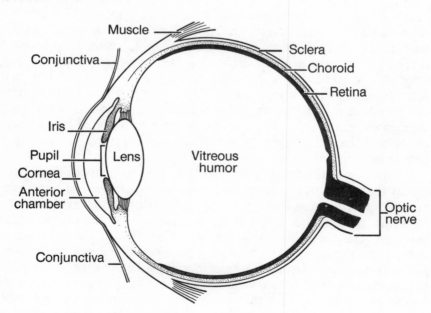

Glaucoma

Glaucoma is a condition in which the fluid normally produced inside the eyeball does not drain through its normal drainage channels as quickly as it is supposed to. The pressure that the excess fluid produces increases and presses on the optic nerve. If the pressure remains elevated for a period of time it will damage the optic nerve, initially causing a loss of some peripheral vision but eventually (if the condition remains untreated) leading to complete blindness.

Cataracts

The clear lens of the eye is formed of transparent proteins whose chemical structure can change. The lens is often described by analogy to an egg white: it can be transformed from clear to opaque, becoming less flexible as we age. When opacity or cloudiness is seen by an examining eyecare specialist, the condition is called a *cataract*. Contrary to various common beliefs, a cataract is not a film over the eye or a growth inside the eye but a change in the structure of the lens. Three major types of cataracts are likely to occur in older people: nuclear cataracts, which occur in the nucleus of the lens; cortical cataracts, which arise in the surrounding cortex; and posterior subcapsular cataracts, which develop in front of the posterior capsule of the lens. If the cataract forms in the line of sight, vision may become blurred or foggy, and things may no longer appear as bright as they once did. At an advanced stage, the entire lens may be so cloudy that it is actually opaque, severely impairing vision. If the cataract continues to advance and surgery is not performed, blindness will ensue. Worldwide, approximately 17 million people are blinded by cataracts (because of lack of surgery), making this condition the leading cause of blindness in the world.

Cataracts constitute the most common eye problem afflicting people in their later years. It is estimated that 90 percent of sixty-five-year-old people show some signs of cataract formation in their eyes, although their vision may not be impaired. And because it often develops very gradually, eyesight may not be affected for many years, if ever. If a person's vision becomes so limited that he or she cannot perform normal activities, the person will probably want to have the cataract removed. Cataract surgery today is a routine procedure that is reasonably safe even for the very elderly. While it still has risks, the surgery has been greatly streamlined. The entire lens may be removed, or just the cataract, leaving the posterior capsule of the lens intact.

Typically, it is not even necessary to remain in the hospital overnight. Eyeglasses, a contact lens, or a synthetic intraocular lens (a substitute for the natural lens that is permanently placed into position during the cataract extraction surgery) provides the individual with improved vision after surgery. More than 1 million cataract operations are performed each year in the United States.

Although cataracts are most often age-related, they can also occur earlier in life. Congenital cataracts may result from a hereditary disorder or from prenatal exposure to harmful influences. Injury to the eye—especially if a wound penetrates the eyeball—can result in the development of a cataract. Diabetics, whether controlled or not, have a three to four times greater chance than other people of forming cataracts. Medically supervised or unsupervised use of certain cortisone or cortisone-like drugs (which are actually steroids) can lead these chemicals to react with the proteins in the lens, forming molecules that accumulate, clouding the lens. Various kinds of radiation can induce the growth of reactive fragments called *free radicals* that cause the lens protein to oxidize, encouraging development of a cataract. A little later we will discuss the specific effect of the sun on the growth of cataracts.

Retinal Disorders

Disorders of the retina are also fairly common among older people. *Macular degeneration* refers to a condition that adversely affects the macula—the high-resolution or fine-tuning part of the retina needed for close work. Certain types of macular degeneration can be treated, but often the lost vision cannot be restored. *Peripheral retinal degeneration* refers to a change in or destruction of tissue at the periphery of the retina. This condition may not itself affect vision, but it can lead to retinal detachment, which occurs when a hole in the retina permits the liquid vitreous humor in the center of the eye to seep behind the retina, pushing it away from the back of the eyeball. Peripheral retinal degeneration can be treated surgically, and if caught early (before it reaches the macula) it has a high rate of success.

Some medical conditions affect the eyes. Diabetes, for instance, in addition to being associated with a higher rate of cataract development, can spur development of diabetic retinopathy, in which damage to the retina is caused by abnormal growth of or leakage from the small blood vessels in the retina of the eye.

Ultraviolet Radiation

As was stated earlier, in order for the eye to fulfill its main function as the sensory organ of vision, light must penetrate the tissues of the eye and reach the retina, where absorption takes place. But ultraviolet radiation, whether incurred from the sun or in tanning salons, can have very deleterious effects upon the eyes.

What are some of the specific hazards? Most people have noticed a feeling of discomfort and fatigue from driving, fishing, skiing, reading or even just casually sitting in glaring sunshine. There are two kinds of glare that you may have experienced. When the sun is extremely bright and the overall level of light is very high, you may experience direct glare. Reflected glare occurs when concentrated light bounces off a white or shiny surface, such as water or snow.

As chapter 1 noted, the types of energy that are emitted from the sun include radio waves, X rays, infrared rays, visible light, and ultraviolet radiation. Infrared rays, which provide much of the heat on our planet, are not considered harmful, but in combination with wind they can cause the natural moisture in the eyes to dry out. Most of our concern in this book, however, focuses on ultraviolet radiation—especially UV-A and UV-B. UV-C is absorbed in the upper atmosphere, but UV-A and UV-B reach the surface of the earth, where UV-A represents 5.5 percent of total solar energy and UV-B represents only 0.5 percent. UV-A can induce sunburn, but not nearly as intensely as UV-B; however, it penetrates through three layers of skin and causes long-term damage, including wrinkles and cancer of the skin. UV-B penetrates only the first two layers, but its intensity enables it to cause both immediate and long-term damage. The depletion of the fragile and protective ozone layer, a consequence of artificially prepared chemicals that have been released into the atmosphere, permits much more ultraviolet radiation to reach the earth than in previous times, thus increasing our risk of damage from the sun.

The Sun and Eyes

Does ultraviolet radiation affect the eyes? It certainly does. Sometimes eyes are already contaminated with a virus that hasn't yet evidenced itself. Some studies indicate that there is a higher rate of such infections—including conjunctivitis—requiring treatment after exposure to sunlight.

Sunburn of the eyelids doesn't usually occur, because the eyelids normally move, but a person who falls asleep in the sun may discover that the lids have become seriously sunburned, with accompanying pain and swelling. And individuals with a history of prolonged sun exposure are at risk of basal cell and squamous cell cancers and malignant melanoma of the eyelid. These cancers are discussed in chapters 7 and 8.

Reflexes make people blink and squint in strong sunlight, and these reactions offer some protection to the eyes. The cornea also reflects and absorbs some UVR; and although some damage to it may occur, the cornea repairs itself quickly. Moreover, its action serves to prevent some permanent damage to the eye. There is speculation that the present-day increase in exposure attributable to the thinning of the protective ozone layer may result in long-range permanent damage to the cornea. The lens of the eye also absorbs some of the light, and because it yellows with age, its capacity to absorb light increases with age. But while it absorbs the UVR not already intercepted by the cornea, it also places itself at risk of developing cataracts. People who have had all or part of a lens removed (for treatment of cataracts) no longer have this protection and must take special precautions to guard their eyes against ultraviolet radiation. However, some intraocular lens (placed after cataract surgery) contain compounds that absorb UV light. Currently, most lenses offer this protection, but some opthalmologists prefer not to use such lenses. If you are planning cataract surgery, discuss this with the ophthalmologist who is doing the procedure. If you have already had cataract surgery, ask the surgeon if a UV-absorbent lens was implanted; they are a fairly recent development.

UVR and the Conjunctiva

Exposure to considerable ultraviolet radiation can cause benign growths on or a thickening of the conjunctiva, the protective membrane that lines the eyelids and covers the eyeball. This, in turn, can result in the appearance of a yellow spot on either side of the cornea— a condition called *pinguecula* that can be unsightly. Finally, pinguecula can lead to pterygia—the formation of a thick, triangular bit of pale tissue that extends from the border of the cornea near the nose toward the middle of the eye. Pterygia can also result directly from ultraviolet radiation; it is fairly common in some equatorial climates, as the physiological result of a hot, dry climate and nearly vertical rays of sunlight.

Cancer of the conjunctiva, although rare, has been associated with prolonged sun exposure. According to the Skin Cancer Foundation, such problems are more likely to occur in people who live close to the equator, where the sun is strongest, or who pursue outdoor occupations, such as farmers, fishermen, and construction workers.

The cornea blocks much of the ultraviolet radiation that reaches the eye, and the crystalline lens inside the eye prevents almost all of the remaining UVR from reaching the retina. But the effects of UVR— and in particular, UV-B—on the cornea can be very dramatic.

Snow Blindness

The American Academy of Ophthalmology has 16,000 members and is the world's largest organization of eye physicians and surgeons. Members like to advise people on taking care of their eyes, and in the spring of each year they send out warnings about some of the dangers that lurk on the ski slopes. Many skiers believe that spring is the best time of all for skiing, because snow and sun coexist. But this is also the most likely time to develop a severe case of sunburn of the eyes, called *snow blindness*—a temporary but aptly named condition. Surfers too are at great risk of incurring this condition, because the concentrated reflected light from the water has the same effect as does the light from the snow.

Symptoms can be quite frightening: a gritty sensation and conjunctival redness progressing to pain, inability to tolerate any kind of light, and uncontrollable lid closure. Upon examination, the center of the surface of the cornea seems to be denuded of cells, the cause of the intense pain. Generally the condition clears up on its own in a few days, although sometimes lubricants, pain relievers, antibiotics, or patching of the eye is prescribed by an ophthalmologist. Excessive exposure of the delicate tissues in the eye to ultraviolet radiation causes this painful, albeit temporary condition. As one victim said, "I felt as if someone had taken sandpaper and stroked it back and forth against my eye." Anyone who experiences persistent symptoms or a great deal of pain should consult an ophthalmologist.

Snow blindness, medically known as *ultraviolet keratoconjunctivitis*, can easily be prevented by wearing goggles or sunglasses that filter out the ultraviolet radiation produced by the sun. In Part Two we will discuss the best types of sunglasses to use for various activities, including skiing.

Painful though snow blindness may be, there is little evidence that the damage to the cornea is permanent. But damage to the lens of the eye from chronic exposure to the sun is another story!

UVR and Cataract Formation

For many years, ophthalmologists have suspected an association between long exposure to ultraviolet radiation and the formation of cataracts. It had long been noted that people living in areas where there was a great deal of sunshine had a relatively high rate of cataracts. Furthermore, studies in laboratory animals had demonstrated that ultraviolet radiation damaged the animals' lenses.

A major study published in the December 1, 1988, *New England Journal of Medicine* and conducted by Hugh R. Taylor, MD, and his colleagues at the Johns Hopkins School of Medicine in Baltimore indicated that extensive exposure to sunlight can triple a person's risk of developing a cortical cataract, the type of cataract that forms in the outer layer of the lens.

The study involved a survey of 838 Chesapeake Bay watermen, ranging in age and in the number of years they had worked on the bay. Dr. Taylor and his staff chose this group because they formed a stable occupational group with a varied amount of total sun exposure. The study combined a very detailed occupational history of each man from the age of 16, laboratory and field measurements that revealed how much sun each man had been exposed to, and ophthalmological examinations to determine the type and extent of any cataracts.

Using sophisticated mathematical measures, Dr. Taylor and his group were able to demonstrate conclusively that the men who had developed cortical cataracts had been exposed to much more UV-B from the age of 16 onward than had those who hadn't developed this type of cataract. UV-B, you will recall, is the type of radiation that causes severe sunburns, and it is more clearly implicated in skin cancers than UV-A is. Although far less UV-B than UV-A reaches the earth (it is highest in summer and in the tropics between 10 A.M. and 2 P.M.), many scientists believe that the amounts of it penetrating the earth's atmosphere are increasing because of the deterioration of the protective ozone layer. Dr. Taylor estimates that, for every 10 percent increase in UV-B, there will be a 6 percent increase in cortical cataracts.

Unlike epidermal skin color, which has a significant affect on how a person's skin reacts to the sun, iris color does not seem to make any difference in a person's level of protection from UV-related eye problems. So whether your eyes are light blue or dark brown, excessive exposure to UV-B puts you in the same high-risk category for developing cataracts. Individuals who have had a cataract removed need to be mindful that their eyes are especially vulnerable to damage by the sun, unless an intraocular lens containing UV-absorbent compounds was implanted.

UVR and the Retina

According to many researchers, years of exposure to ultraviolet radiation may seriously damage the retina, resulting in age-related macular degeneration. Some studies have found no connection between exposure to ultraviolet radiation and the later development of macular degeneration, but other research suggests that a link exists. And related studies have indicated that intense light can cause retinal damage in monkeys.

Paul Sternberg, Jr., MD, assistant professor of ophthalmology at Emory University in Atlanta, and other investigators concerned about the potential danger of ultraviolet radiation to the retina have searched for ways to protect it from injury. Their work is based on the theory that the retina is jeopardized by oxidative damage to the retinal pigment epithelium (one of its layers). But until some way of medically protecting the retina from damage is perfected, it is perhaps wisest to rely on UV-protective sunglasses and a brimmed hat. Given that macular degeneration affects 28 percent of people seventy-five to eighty-five years of age and that over 100,000 Americans are legally blind as a result of it, you should certainly be cautious about spending much time in the sun without protecting your eyes.

Photosensitivity

In earlier chapters we discussed photosensitivity—the occurrence of adverse skin reactions following exposure to both UVR and certain medications or chemicals. People who are taking medication internally or who suffer from a disease that causes photosensitivity need to be especially protective of their eyes in the sun, since ocular damage has also been associated with photosensitivity. Anyone undergoing PUVA treatment (in which a photosensitive drug called Psoralen is administered to the patient, and then a particular area of the patient is exposed under medical care to ultraviolet radiation) for psoriasis or some other condition must take care to protect eyes and skin when sun exposure cannot be avoided.

Tanning Devices

In the spring of 1989, the Centers for Disease Control of the U.S. Department of Health and Human Services reported on a study done in Wisconsin, where dermatologists, ophthalmologists, and emergency-room personnel were surveyed about injuries caused by tanning devices. The 48 ophthalmologists who completed the questionnaire had treated a total of 162 patients during the preceding year for eye injuries related to tanning devices. Of these patients, 129 had suffered corneal injuries, 4 had suffered both corneal and retinal injuries, and 19 had suffered unspecified eye injuries.

Why didn't these tanning enthusiasts wear safety goggles? Many of them did: 24 percent of those who sustained eye injuries from suntanning devices were wearing safety goggles during the tanning session. In these cases, either some radiation seeped through or around the goggles or the goggles themselves did not totally block out the rays.

Brandford L. Walters, MD, and Ted Martin Kelley, MD, from Michigan State University commented in an article in the *American Journal of Emergency Medicine* that it used to be rare for emergency-room physicians to see instances of burns to the cornea, and when they did the burns were usually the result of accidental exposure to chemical or physical agents. For example, people involved in heavy industrial manufacturing might be burned by arc welders. Occasionally the burn might be caused by a home sunlamp or by direct exposure to the sun while sunbathing or boating.

The study conducted by Dr. Walters and Dr. Kelley found that the incidence of corneal burns had increased greatly in the mid-1980s. Of the patients treated at two different emergency rooms for UV-light-induced corneal burns, 40 percent had been exposed at a commercial tanning facility. The researchers noted that the number of corneal burns increased as more commercial tanning facilities began sprouting up around Michigan State University. Many of the people who turned up in emergency rooms for treatment of corneal burns had completed a session under the UV lights just a few hours earlier. Most of the burns were not serious and healed with little or no treatment. But not everyone was so lucky. After exposure to tanning devices, two people noticed blind spots that didn't go away. When they saw an ophthalmologist a few days later, they were informed that severe burns had occurred on their retinas; both individuals were left with substantial permanent loss of vision.

In chapter 3 we discussed tanning devices in some depth. Dermatologists are in agreement that even devices promoted by their manufacturers as "safe UVA" units are *not* safe. Ophthalmologists concur: the wise policy is to stay away from them. But if you insist on using any type of sunlamp or tanning bed, be sure to protect your eyes with goggles that are sanitized (otherwise they can transmit eye infections from the previous user) and that fit tightly. Closing your eyes will not protect them; both solar UVR and artificially produced UVR can sear right through your eyelids.

Cancer and Eyes

The cumulative effect of exposure to the sun has been linked conclusively to skin cancer, and most people associate these cancers with lesions on the face, hands, or other frequently exposed areas of the body. Malignant melanoma, which may occur on exposed or unexposed areas of the body, is usually found in individuals who have had intermittent sun exposure or a history of searing sunburns during childhood. These life-threatening cancers can also occur on the eyelid, and if detected early can be treated very successfully. Unfortunately, when they are allowed to progress to an advanced stage before diagnosis, extensive surgery may be necessary. Melanoma can also develop inside the eye. In chapters 7 and 8, we will discuss cancers of the skin and eyes and treatments for them.

Protecting Yourself

Sunglasses are a must on any day that is sunny enough to give you a sunburn. A brimmed hat or billed baseball-type cap can cut sun exposure of the eyes by one-quarter to one-half and thus is a wise investment. Dr. Jacqueline Lustgarten of the Mount Sinai School of Medicine is as careful about summer sun as she is about the ski slopes.

She urges her patients to take sensible precautions, and sends her sons off to camp each day with sunscreen, sunglasses, and a baseball cap. In Part Two of this book, where we discuss protection from the sun, we will investigate how to choose appropriate sunglasses.

Summary

The eye, our sensory organ of vision, is a complex structure. Problems with the eyes and vision can be minor, requiring corrective glasses, or serious enough to warrant surgery. Sometimes conditions due to sunburn or other causes are not reversible, and vision is lost. Scientific studies indicate that ultraviolet radiation can affect many parts of the eye: the cornea can be seriously burned; snow blindness, though temporary, can be very painful; the retina may be damaged; sometimes permanently; the conjunctiva can thicken; and cataract formation is closely linked with cumulative exposure to UV-B. In addition, people who are photosensitive for any reason may suffer ocular damage as a result of the condition. A number of serious (and sometimes irreversible) accidents have been reported as a result of protected or unprotected exposure to sunlamps or other tanning devices.

Cancers of the eyelids and melanoma of the eye itself or of the eyelid are closely associated with UVR exposure. Protecting your eyes from ultraviolet radiation is not complicated: appropriate sunglasses and a hat with a visor can markedly reduce the potential for damage.

7   *Cancer of the Skin*

"It's only skin cancer." How many times have you heard people say that? Whether they are breathing a sigh of relief that they don't have a life-threatening form of cancer or they are trying to console a friend who has been given a recent diagnosis, the average person tends to perceive skin cancer as a minor problem. It's true that most skin cancers are curable, but they can still be serious and sometimes disfiguring. The American Cancer Society estimates that 50 percent of all people who live to the age of sixty-five will have at least one. And over 2,000 people die each year of nonmelanoma skin cancers. Even malignant melanoma—if caught early—is curable, as we will discuss in chapter 8.

What Is Cancer?

Cancer is a general term used to describe various groups of diseases characterized by abnormal cell growth in the body. Cancer cells do not usually stay in any one place; instead they move around, crowding between normal cells and even penetrating them. Unchecked by medical intervention, these cells tend to spread to distant body sites.

Cancer cells differ from normal cells in many ways. They have an irregular, disordered appearance when viewed under a microscope; they serve no useful function in the body; and they do not wear out and die. Instead, these malignant cells continually divide and multiply, reproducing themselves as they invade and destroy surrounding tissues.

Cancer is not just one disease but many related diseases. It can arise in any organ or tissue of the body. In this book we will concern ourselves only with cancers that arise on the skin and whose cell growth begins in one or more layers of the skin. The major types of skin cancers are basal cell and squamous cell carcinomas (a carcinoma is a type of cancer that grows in tissue that covers or lines the body or internal organs), and malignant melanoma. Malignant melanoma is a life-threatening illness because the melanoma cancer cells can metastasize (spread) throughout the body.

You will remember from our discussion in chapter 2 that the skin is the body's largest organ. The visible portion of the skin, called the *epidermis,* consists of several different cell types and layers of cells. The bottom row of cells is composed of basal cells; the middle layer consists of squamous cells. Melanin-producing melanocytes are interspersed between them. Squamous cells are fast-growing cells that have matured and moved upward from the basal layer. If basal cells become cancerous, the growth or lesion is called a *basal cell carcinoma;* if squamous cells become cancerous, the condition is called *squamous cell carcinoma.* When melanocytes become malignant, the result is *melanoma.*

Is Skin Cancer Common?

More than ½ million new cases of skin cancer are diagnosed in the United States each year. That represents one-third of all new cancers. It is predicted that one in seven Americans will develop skin cancer in his or her lifetime. The rates in other parts of the world are comparable. Among Caucasians alive today, the risk of developing nonmelanoma skin cancer is about 30 percent; and among those born after 1985, the lifetime risk of developing it is about 40 percent.

As evidence that skin cancer is caused by sun exposure, 90 percent of all skin cancers occur on parts of the body that have been exposed to the sun, among people who spend long hours in the sun. According to the Skin Cancer Foundation, skin cancer takes decades to develop, and the effects of ultraviolet radiation are cumulative. Thus, even a few weeks of sunbathing each summer will, after twenty or more years, amount to considerable exposure, which in vulnerable people could lead to skin cancer.

Who Is at Greatest Risk of Getting Skin Cancer?

People with the least melanin in their skin—those with Type 1 or Type 2 skin (fair skin and blue or green eyes), as described in the chart on page 000—are especially susceptible to developing skin cancer. In addition, people who have been exposed to radiation from X rays, chemicals such as coal tars and arsenic (at one time used to treat various diseases, including asthma), thermal burns, and chronic draining of the sinuses have an unusually high vulnerability.

Since skin cancer takes years to develop, people with the largest amount of cumulative exposure to UVR are the ones at greatest risk.

Melanoma, which we will discuss in the next chapter, is related to episodes of burning and to short intensive exposures. Exhaustive studies have shown that the people most likely to get skin cancer belong to one or more of the following groups:

* Those who have fair skin and sunburn easily (Type 1 or 2 skin)
* Those who are photosensitive
* Those who live in the south or southwest United States or in other areas of the world relatively near the equator (the number of cases doubles with every 8 degrees latitude nearer the equator)
* Those who live at high altitudes (more UVB light penetrates the thinner atmosphere; the city with the highest rate of skin cancer in the United States is Albuquerque, New Mexico, where the altitude is high and the latitude is low)
* Those who experience prolonged exposure to the sun, such as:
  construction workers
  farmers
  athletes (professional and amateur)
  sailors and others who work on the water
  lifeguards
  ski instructors
  sun-worshipers
* Those with genetic conditions predisposing them to skin cancer (such as Gorlin's syndrome, xeroderma pigmentosa, or albinism)
* Those with excessive exposure to X rays
* Relatives of people who have had basal cell carcinomas
* Men, more than women, in the over-forty age range
* Women, more than men, in the under-forty age range
* Those who have a number of unusual moles
* Those who have had severe childhood or adolescent sunburns
* Those whose families have a history of melanoma

People who fall into one or more of the above categories are at highest risk, but everyone—with the exception of most dark-skinned African-Americans—is at risk of developing skin cancer as a result of continued, unprotected exposure to the sun.

The Skin Cancer Foundation states that 80 percent of an individual's lifetime sun exposure is received by the age of twenty; thus, for many adults, protection from the sun may not be enough. They must be aware of the warning signs of skin cancer so that it can be diagnosed and treated early, when a cure is easily obtained.

Who Actually Develops Skin Cancer?

Individuals in the highest risk categories are the most likely to develop cancer, but anyone can get it. Twice as many men as women get skin cancer, but the difference in rates may be related to the greater numbers of men who have traditionally worked in outdoor occupations. As more women enter fields such as police, construction, and sports or spend their leisure time on the tennis courts or golf course, the rates are likely to change. Indeed, they are already changing in geographical areas where there is lots of sun; and some studies indicate that, before age forty, more women than men develop skin cancer.

Unfortunately, people subject to considerable sun exposure where the sun is hottest and the altitude is highest are at great risk even if they don't sunbathe or routinely work outdoors, just in going about their normal activities of daily living without using sunscreens and other forms of protection against the sun's rays. Those who spend considerable time in the sun, under almost any geographical conditions, may eventually pay for it by developing skin cancer.

Combine such factors as light skin, long hours in the sun, a high altitude, and low latitude, and—even if you do escape skin cancer—your skin will suffer significant damage.

Some diseases and genetic conditions predispose people to develop skin cancer. These include xeroderma pigmentosa, xeroderma, Gorlin's syndrome, and albinism.

Xeroderma pigmentosa: This rare, inherited skin disease is characterized by sensitivity to UVR; exposure to UVR results in freckles, keratoses, and skin cancers. The condition usually starts in childhood, and most people who have it are unable to repair skin normally following exposure to UVR. The skin of affected people shows early aging (even before age five). Frequently, skin cancer develops in these individuals.

Xeroderma: This chronic inherited skin condition is characterized by irregularly pigmented skin that first appears extremely dry and rough and later becomes thin, ulcerated, and scarred. Even brief exposure to the sun exacerbates these conditions and can lead to cancer.

Gorlin's syndrome: This rare genetic condition renders people susceptible to various skin disorders and multiple basal cell carcinomas.

Albinism: This genetic condition places people at special risk of damage from UVR. Born with partial or total lack of melanin pigment, albinos are prone to serious sunburns and to skin cancer. People with total albinism have pale skin, white hair, and pink eyes; they are represented in all ethnic groups.

Where on the Body Does Skin Cancer Usually Occur?

About 80 percent of skin cancers occur on the face, head, or neck; another 10 percent occur on other exposed areas of the body, such as the backs of hands. According to Perry Robbins, MD, associate professor of clinical dermatology at the New York University School of Medicine and founder of the Skin Cancer Foundation, 25 to 35 percent of all skin cancers arise on or around the nose. Another 20 percent of them occur around the eye, many on the eyelids themselves. Skin cancer may develop anywhere on the face (including the lips), on the tips of the ears (especially in men and women whose hair doesn't cover their ears), and on the top of the heads of bald or balding men. Men's shoulders, backs, and chests and women's lower legs have become more common sites in recent years, a result of the last several decades of sun exposure to these locations.

People who drive cars in the United States are more likely to develop a skin cancer lesion on their left arm or the left side of their face than on the right side, because when they drive with open windows their left side is more exposed to the sun. In Great Britain there is a higher incidence of skin cancer on the right side of the face and on the right arm, reflecting the opposite driving sides in the two countries.

What are Premalignant Lesions?

Even before cancer actually occurs on the skin, a premalignant lesion (growth) may appear. In chapter 2 we discussed some of such growths that have the potential to become malignant. Actinic keratoses, sometimes called *solar keratoses,* are appropriately named because they appear almost exclusively on people who have had a great deal of sun exposure. They consist of smooth, flat, or slightly raised pink spots that later become irregular, scaly, and wartlike (actual warts do not become cancerous) and are red or brownish in color. Like skin cancers themselves, they usually develop in exposed areas such as the face or the backs of hands.

These scaly, hyperpigmented lesions were once called *farmer's skin* or *seaman's skin* because they were generally found on people who pursued outdoor occupations. In the past they were most often seen in older people, and since there was a time lag between the development of these lesions and subsequent actual skin cancer, many physicians did not recommend treatment. Today people live longer, and these premalignant lesions are showing up on younger people, so treatment is recommended for almost everyone who develops actinic keratoses.

Some of these premalignant keratoses are known as *senile keratoses,* and they may be found in older people on parts of the body that have not been exposed to sunlight.

Keratoacanthoma is a fast-growing, uncommon skin lesion that most often occurs on sun-exposed areas of the body. Although it invades the skin, it does not spread and can clear up without treatment. It usually appears as a smooth, red nodule, often with an umbilical spot in the center. It can be aggressive and locally destructive of skin tissue.

Leukoplakia is a precancerous condition that generally appears in mucous membranes on the lips or on the inside of the mouth. The symptomatic smooth, opaque white patches are associated with pipe smoking.

In Part Three of this book, we will discuss a wide range of treatments for both precancers and cancers.

Is It Cancer?

Only a physician can tell for sure whether a particular growth is cancerous or not. But you can check a number of things yourself. Perhaps a good simple rule to remember is this:

If a new growth or discoloration appears and doesn't go away after a few weeks, or if a change (in color, size, shape, or thickness) occurs in an existing mole, growth, or discoloration, see a doctor.

The American Cancer Society, the American Academy of Dermatology, and the Skin Cancer Foundation all urge you to perform regular self-examinations of your skin. This will enable you to detect the beginnings of any skin cancer—including the most serious one, malignant melanoma, which will be described in full in chapter 8.

In a well-lit room, use a full-length mirror and a small mirror to examine more difficult-to-see places. With a hair brush or (even better) a blow dryer for pushing away your hair to see your scalp, examine *all* of your skin, looking for the following warning signs:

* An existing pimple, growth, small sore, or other lesion that
  — hasn't healed
  — is getting larger
  — looks irritated
  — itches, scabs, or bleeds
* A pale, waxy, pearly looking lump that
  — suddenly appears
  — becomes an open sore
* A red, scaly, sharply outlined patch of skin
* An existing mole that
  — changes in size
  — becomes red, white, or partially blue or has other tiny dark spots
  — begins to bleed
  — becomes darker in color
* New moles—especially if colored a uniform bluish black or bluish gray or exhibiting an uneven surface

An untrained eye can only detect so much! As an experienced health writer, I readily understand and can clearly describe medical information; but I'm not trained to observe and as a result I have been known to overreact to medical problems within my family. In fact, our personal physician, internist Stephen P. Nachtigall, MD, of Fresh Meadows, New York, says he can always tell what I'm currently researching or writing about by the nature of the medical concerns I express for either my husband or myself. While I was working on this book, I sent my husband off to the doctor to examine a "growth," as I described it, on his lower leg. I was sure that it was skin cancer, but rather than alarm him I said reassuringly, "It's probably just a little reaction from an insect bite."

He returned from the dermatologist, impressed by my diagnosis. It turned out to have been exactly what I said—not, fortunately, what I really thought. The doctor gave him some ointment, which cleared it up quickly, and it didn't recur, confirming that it wasn't anything very serious.

This story illustrates how easy it is to fall into the habit of trying to diagnose our own medical conditions and either overreacting (which at the worst costs time and money) or underreacting (which can cost you your well-being and even your life). The best course, whenever you are in doubt, is to see your personal physician first and then, if symptoms persist, to see a dermatologist. Appendix II includes a section explaining how to find a dermatologist.

The Dermatologist's Examination

If you're lucky, the suspected skin cancer you bring to the attention of a dermatologist will be diagnosed as a temporary or even self-limiting condition (something that goes away on its own), and you will be relieved to know that you don't have cancer.

When you first visit the dermatologist, you will be asked some relevant questions about your own personal and family medical history. You may wish to think about this ahead of time and be prepared to answer these questions:

* Have you ever had any form of skin cancer?
* Has a physician ever told you that you had a skin precancer?
* Are you or were you at one time regularly exposed to sun at work or leisure?
* Do you protect yourself from the sun with sunscreen or protective clothing? When did you begin to do this?
* Does anyone in your family have a number of moles?
* Has anyone in your family had basal cell or squamous cell skin cancer?
* Has anyone in your family ever had melanoma?
* When did you first notice the sore or spot you are here to have examined?
* Has it changed since then? If so, how?

The dermatologist will then examine the area. His or her trained eye—aided by nothing more than a magnifying glass—can sometimes determine that a growth is completely harmless. But before sending you on your way, reassured, praised for your caution, and reminded to return if any changes in the growth occur or any new ones appear, the dermatologist is likely to do a total body skin exam.

As Deborah S. Sarnoff, MD, a dermatologist at the New York University Medical Center, explained in an article in the 1986 *Journal of the Skin Cancer Foundation,* a total body skin examination involves a thorough inspection of your skin by a physician who is a trained skin specialist. This procedure is performed to determine whether any abnormality exists in your skin, hair, or nails. In a well-lighted examining room, the physician will carefully examine all areas of your skin, including not-so-visible parts such as your scalp and the backs of your ears.

The Skin Cancer Foundation, the American Academy of Dermatology, and the American Cancer Society recommend that *everyone* have a total body skin examination (TBSE) once a year. If you fall into a high-risk category because of skin type, history of sun-exposure, *and* either a tendency toward unusual or numerous moles or a family history of skin cancer, you may even arrange to have such examinations more frequently. If you have had any precancerous lesions as described in chapter 2, you should be examined by a dermatologist regularly and frequently. Your physician can also aid you in learning more about self-examination.

Why should everyone have a TBSE annually? Dr. Sarnoff offers three good reasons:

* You may have an abnormal mole where you can't easily see it, such as on your back.
* You may not recognize a premalignant growth as significant.
* Skin sometimes serves as a window for diagnosing other diseases, such as thyroid conditions, internal cancers, or diabetes. A thorough examination of the skin may aid in early detection of these conditions.

Although many dermatologists and family doctors routinely advise patients to have a TBSE, others only recommend this for patients who have a personal history of skin cancer. Dr. Sarnoff suggests that you ask your dermatologist (or make an appointment with one especially for this purpose) to perform this examination. It only takes a few minutes, and the examination is usually included in the cost of a regular office visit.

Suspect Growths

Even the most experienced dermatologist can't always be certain that a benign (noncancerous) growth really is benign. Sometimes the most highly trained eye and most powerful magnifying glass cannot, with absolute certainty, determine a diagnosis. In such an instance, the dermatologist may recommend a biopsy.

By definition, a *biopsy* is the removal and microscopic examination of suspect tissue or body fluid. Properly performed, it can provide the definitive diagnosis of cancer; and in all instances it should be done by a physician who is well trained and experienced so that sufficient tissue is removed for examination. Preparation and examination of the biopsied tissue are equally important, and these duties are the responsibility of both the physician and the pathologist (a physician specially trained to study and evaluate the characteristics, causes, and effects of disease through the use of laboratory tests and other methods). At this time, before or after biopsy, you may wish to seek a second opinion.

Although different types of biopsies are performed, depending on the nature of the suspect internal or external growth, the type of biopsy done on skin lesions is usually described as a curettage or as an incisional or excisional biopsy. This is a surgical procedure, usually done in the doctor's office or in a hospital outpatient operating room. During the procedure, the mole, small lump, or growth is removed in part or (if it is small) in its entirety, and then submitted to a pathologist for examination.

Biopsies are not all the same. An incisional biopsy, in which a small piece (rather than the entire growth) is removed, is often performed on a suspected growth of skin cancer. The method used to achieve this varies according to the type of growth. Among the possibilities are the following:

* *Shave biopsy:* Tissue is thinly sliced off with a scalpel.
* *Curette or scrape biopsy:* Tissue is superficially scraped off.
* *Scissor biopsy:* A growth that protrudes above the surface of skin is removed.
* *Sponge biopsy:* A lesion is abraded with a cellulose sponge.
* *Wedge biopsy:* A preshaped portion is excised.
* *Punch biopsy:* A small piece of tissue is removed, using a special instrument (something like a cookie cutter) or a scalpel that pierces through the skin to remove a deeper part of growth. This

method is used when growth itself is too large to remove merely for diagnostic purposes. Generally, stitches are required to close the skin following this kind of biopsy.

In many instances, the entire growth is removed in a procedure termed an *excisional biopsy*. This is done when the growth is small or when it is essential to know the extent and depth of the suspected cancer.

If the pathologist finds the sample noncancerous, you will have a good reason to celebrate but not to relax, since you will want to remain vigilant for any subsequent growths.

If the biopsy report is positive for cancer, your doctor will identify what kind of cancer it is, tell whether it has spread to the outer borders of the sample, and outline any treatment recommendations. Before proceeding with treatment, you may wish to seek a second opinion, if you have not yet done so; your insurance company may even insist upon this. Treatments will be described in Part Three.

Because at least 10 percent of all individuals with newly diagnosed skin cancers have more than one skin cancer at the same time, the dermatologist will be especially careful to examine your entire body, even if you only consulted the doctor for only one growth. Your lymph nodes near the suspected malignancy will also be examined to determine whether they are enlarged.

Basal Cell Carcinoma

Slow growing but potentially destructive, basal cell carcinoma is the most common of all cancers, including skin cancers. Sometimes referred to as *basal cell epitheliomas*, these cancerous growths affect more than 400,000 people yearly. They grow out of the cells in the deep basal layer of the epidermis and are seen most often on individuals with white skin—particularly people of North European extraction. Basal cell carcinoma (BCC) does not metastasize (spread), as internal cancers do, but if left untreated it can badly damage and destroy underlying tissues and structures. If neglected, BCC around the eyes or ears can lead to disfigurement and even loss of function of these organs.

BCC usually begins on a sun-exposed area of the body: the face, ears, neck, scalp, shoulders, or back. The tumors may also begin on nonexposed areas.

At one time, BCC usually struck older people, especially men who had worked outdoors; it was seldom seen in children, teenagers, and people in their twenties. Today, however, the incidence has increased markedly among males and females in these age groups, as well as among those in midlife. No one is immune to it.

In almost every instance, the onset of BCC is directly related to sun exposure. Exceptions involve exposure to arsenic or radiation and complications resulting from burns, scars, vaccinations, or tattoos. Of course, these factors can also contribute to the onset of BCC that is primarily sun-related.

A number of warning signs are specific for BCC. Appearance of the cancer usually can be felt as well as seen, and the growth may have pearly or shiny edges. The color may be reddish or purplish and may even have small red dots around it. In dark-skinned people, the bump can be so dark that it looks like a mole.

An open sore that is at first mistaken for an insect bite or scratch that doesn't heal and/or begins to bleed, ooze, or crust can often be a sign of BCC. Basal cell carcinomas are still sometimes referred to as *rodent ulcers,* because of their resemblance to a rat bite—a once-common phenomenon.

Sometimes a reddish patch or irritated area on the chest, shoulders, arms, or legs may persist, itch, hurt, or crust. The growth may be smooth with an indentation in the center that may slowly enlarge, with tiny blood vessels developing on the surface. Less often, BCC may first appear as a pale or waxy area on taut skin, resembling a scar without sharp borders.

If you find these symptoms a bit confusing, you are not alone. BCC has many variations in size, shape, and color, and it can mask itself as anything from a cyst to a scar to a sore to a bite; thus, it is quite difficult, if not impossible, for a nonphysician to self-diagnose.

William T. Keavy, MD, in the 1989 *Journal of the Skin Cancer Foundation,* says it best: "this capricious lesion takes on many forms. And that means that when one notices something unusual, especially on those parts of the body that are normally exposed to sunlight, it should be brought to the attention of a physician who can then take the necessary steps towards diagnosis and treatment."

When you see a dermatologist, he or she will establish a diagnosis (if the growth is suspicious) by means of a biopsy and will then determine the best method of treatment. If the cancer is identified early, the treatment can easily be administered, often by surgically removing the lesion and allowing normal healing to occur. When BCC has progressed or is in an area near the nose or eyes, however, additional steps—sometimes including skin grafts—may be indicated. In Part Three we will discuss the available treatments.

Squamous Cell Carcinoma

The second most common type of skin cancer, squamous cell carcinoma affects between 80,000 and 100,000 people each year and accounts for about 20 percent of all skin cancers. These cancers not only grow faster than BCC, but they have far greater potential to invade and destroy underlying structures and to metastasize to lymph glands and other parts of the body. Between 1,500 and 2,000 people die each year from squamous cell carcinoma (SCC); but 95 percent of all SCC can be cured if detected and treated early.

SCC most often arises on the rim of the ear, the face, the lips or mouth, or the back of the hand. Usually SCC begins as a slightly raised pink opaque papule or as a red scaly patch or wartlike growth, later ulcerating in the center. The affected area may increase in size, even to the extent of becoming mushroomlike in appearance, crusting and ulcerating in the center.

As with BCC, a high proportion of SCC arises on sun-exposed areas of skin. The cancers may also develop in scar tissue, in areas of chronic irritation, in nonhealing wounds or trauma, in ulcerations, in infections, and in areas of prior radiation treatment. Cases of SCC that arise from causes other than sun exposure are more likely to involve metastasis.

Good sense dictates that anyone who has scars on sun-exposed areas of the body—for instance, on the chest from cardiac surgery— or who has had radiation treatments to the head and neck area, should be especially careful in the sun.

Like BCC, SCC is difficult (particularly in the early stages) for a nonphysician to self-diagnose. Frequent skin self-examinations of all sun-exposed areas, with special attention to areas that have suffered trauma or been exposed to X-rays, are a wise investment of time in skin health and the prevention of cancer growth. Squamous cell carcinoma can be treated successfully, especially at an early stage. Report any changes in skin growths or appearance to a physician, who can make a definitive diagnosis and outline a treatment plan.

Bowen's Disease

Bowen's disease is sometimes described as a precancerous condition, but other experts consider it a rare form of cancer. It appears as a scaling, reddish pink, raised growth, usually on unexposed areas of the skin. Many people with Bowen's disease have taken patent medicines that contain arsenic, such as tonics or appetite stimulants. Skin affected by Bowen's disease may look like a solar keratosis, but the growth becomes large and thick and generally remains within the confines of the epidermis. Also called *intraepidermal epitheliomas,* these growths can become very unsightly and can break out from the epidermis to invade deeper layers of skin, becoming SCC.

Eyelid Cancers

Any cancer that can appear on the rest of the skin can also develop on the eyelid. This sensitive part of the skin is very vulnerable to the sun, and unless you have had a lifetime of protection via sunglasses and a brimmed hat or visor you are vulnerable to it. You need both a hat and glasses, because a hat alone will not protect you from solar radiation that is reflected up from the ground, particularly ground covered by snow or water.

As elsewhere on the body, the most common cancer of the eyelid is BCC, which represents about 80 percent of all eyelid cancers. Most often it appears on the lower lid, but it also occurs on the upper lid, especially among people who have had a long history of sun exposure. SCC accounts for 7 to 9 percent of eyelid tumors, and these too are closely associated with prolonged exposure to UVR. Malignant melanoma, which will be discussed in chapter 8, is also found on eyelids.

Regular ophthalmological examinations provide a good opportunity to detect eyelid cancers. Unlike the rest of your skin, both sides of an eyelid lesion can be examined. Reported cancers of the eyelid in the United States have doubled since 1977. People who live in sunny areas are most at risk.

Eyelid cancers do not always begin, as one might expect, with a lesion. Instead, the earliest sign may be loss of eyelashes, a persistent eye infection, a bump that could be mistaken for a sty, or a bump that goes away and then returns in the same location. Thus, individuals suffering from any of these symptoms should not ignore it or try to treat it themselves, but should see an ophthalmologist, who may perform an office biopsy through the eyelid to examine all layers.

Generally eyelid cancers don't invade the eye, but if a cancerous basal cell hits the globe of the eye, vision is affected and the eye may even have to be removed. Some cancers of the eye can spread to distant areas.

Squamous cell carcinomas of the eyelid can start out as primary lesions or develop from precancerous actinic keratoses. Malignant melanomas can also arise on the outer lining of the eye. The most common eyelid cancers are those of the sebaceous or tear glands, which can recur, invade, and damage the eye itself, and even spread to distant areas. This type of cancer tends to be recognized late because it initially resembles a sty. It should be made clear that most people with sties don't have cancer; but if a sty stubbornly recurs after healing, it should be investigated carefully.

At the spring 1989 Skin Cancer Foundation news conference, Richard Lisman, MD, co-chief of ophthalmic plastic surgery at the Manhattan Eye and Ear Hospital in New York, stated that a very rare but aggressive cancer, sebaceous carcinoma, which may begin in the glands or skin of the eyebrow, is capable of spreading through the lymph system and bloodstream toward the eye, damaging vision and even leading to eye loss. "Cancers of the conjunctiva may be visible as a growth or even an ordinary red eye, accompanied by a chronic discharge," says Dr. Lisman. "These types of cancers may be at an advanced stage or a growth of a skin cancer that originated in the periorbital area [the area around the eye]."

Sometimes redness can harbor a "quiet" cancer of the eyelids. A "misdirected" eyelash should raise suspicions of a chronic infection or a benign, precancerous, or malignant tumor, according to Dr. Lisman. Though many eyelid cancers occur later in life, when prolonged and cumulative sun damage has already occurred, younger people should also be aware of the signs and symptoms. Dr. Lisman explains, "People who in the past would have lost some degree of vision or even their entire eye following the growth of an eyelid cancer can be better treated through early recognition."

Cancer of the eyelids, like most cancers, responds best to treatment when detected early. Treatments for these cancers are surveyed in Part Three.

Does One Skin Cancer Increase the Risk of Getting Another?

In a 1987 article in *Cancer* magazine, June K. Robinson, MD, dermatologist at Northwestern University Medical School in Chicago, reported on a study of 1,000 people who had been diagnosed with a single basal cell carcinoma; of these, 36 percent developed a second one. The most important risk factors were those that initially placed people at risk: a skin complexion that burns instead of tanning (Type 1 or 2 skin), and frequent sun exposure. Dr. Robinson found no significant association between the development of these multiple BCCs and either gender or age.

Leonard H. Goldberg, MD, of Baylor College of Medicine in Houston and his colleagues reported in the 1988 *Journal of the Skin Cancer Foundation* on their own studies to determine which patients are likely to have a recurrence of skin cancer. They discovered that patients developed skin cancers at a faster rate if they were old (risks were progressively higher with increasing age), were male, had more than one skin cancer when initially seen by the dermatologist, and had precancerous lesions.

Every dermatologist with whom I have spoken agrees that all people, regardless of age or sex, should protect themselves from the sun, but most add that those who have already had one cancer need to be especially vigilant because their chances of developing another one are so great; some authorities say their chances of a recurrence are as high as 50 to 60 percent. Most dermatologists recommend that anyone who has had skin cancer be professionally examined two to four times a year.

Malignant Melanoma

Malignant melanoma can begin on the skin, nails, or eye; it is a life-threatening disease that can spread throughout the body. The subject of malignant melanoma will be more fully discussed in chapter 8.

Is Skin Cancer Contagious?

Because close friends or husbands and wives (such as former President and Mrs. Reagan) may both develop the same kind of skin cancer, people often think that it is contagious. However, every scientific study indicates that cancer cannot be contracted from another person. Sharing towels or sunscreens, swimming in the same pool, or being physically intimate with someone who has skin cancer will not give it to you. Exposure to the sun will. All too often, friends, relatives, and married couples share the same hazardous lifestyle, vacationing or working unprotected in the sun.

Summary

Skin cancers such as basal cell carcinoma (BCC) and squamous cell carcinoma (SCC) are not as minor as many people would like to think. Extremely common and increasing each year, these cancers, left unchecked, can invade underlying structures and damage organs such as the eyes and the nose.

The individuals most likely to develop skin cancer are those with fair skin, those who spend considerable time in the sun, and those who have other environmental and genetic vulnerabilities. These cancers usually occur on sun-exposed areas and are often preceded by premalignant lesions.

Existing sores that don't heal and new growths are among the warning signs of skin cancer, but only a physician can determine exactly what particular growths signify. Self-examination of the skin, as well as an examination performed by a dermatologist, should be conducted regularly to ensure early detection and prompt, thorough, and successful treatment. Both BCC and SCC are eminently curable, but in its later stages SCC can metastasize throughout the body, even causing death.

Eyelid cancers are potentially very serious, resulting in the need for significant reconstructive surgery and sometimes in loss of vision. Here, too, protection against UVR and early detection of the cancer play key roles.

8

Malignant Melanoma: The Life-threatening Skin Cancer

Throughout the world, and especially in areas where people have had intense exposure to the sun, the incidence of malignant melanoma is rising at an alarming rate. In the United States it has risen 60 percent in the last thirteen years. In the 1930s it was estimated that a person had a 1 in 1,500 chance of eventually developing malignant melanoma; that rate has now climbed to 1 in 128 chances; and by the year 2000, if the trend continues, 1 out of 90 Caucasians in the United States will develop malignant melanoma. The rates are the same in Canada.

One-third of all new cancers diagnosed each year are skin cancers. One-fifth of these skin cancers are malignant melanomas. Over 27,000 cases of malignant melanoma were diagnosed in the United States during 1989, and the incidence of this cancer is increasing faster (3.4 percent per year) than that of any other cancer, except for lung cancer in women. According to the American Cancer Society and the Skin Cancer Foundation, it now ranks ninth among the top ten types of new cancer cases for all sites, outranking cancer of the pancreas, all leukemias, and stomach cancers.

In 1989 about 6,000 melanoma-related deaths occurred, making melanoma the fourth leading cause of death from cancer among people between the ages of 20 and 50. Despite this grim statistic, melanoma is almost always curable if detected early and treated promptly. Early detection is easily accomplished, since melanoma is visible, in contrast to cancers that begin internally and are difficult to diagnose or even to suspect until they have already spread. For this reason, survival rates are steadily improving, but there remains a pressing need to prevent future cases of melanoma and to teach more people to recognize the early warning signs of the disease so that they can be diagnosed when it is at an early stage.

What is Malignant Melanoma?

Malignant melanoma is a cancer that originates in skin cells called *melanocytes* that are found in the basal layer of the skin. Interestingly, these cells, which produce the dark pigment, melanin, are also found in the respiratory tract and in surrounding nerve cells.

Malignant melanoma develops when melanocytes are transformed into cancer cells—cells that grow abnormally and (in the case of malignant melanoma) migrate to parts of the body far from the original site where they appeared. This movement, called *metastasis*, occurs through the bloodstream or the lymphatic system. Then the cancer cells crowd out other cells, at their new locations, continuing to spread and multiply, reproducing themselves by cell division, invading and destroying surrounding tissues. They may form additional tumors and, by depriving normal cells of nourishment, may cause weight loss and obstruct normal functioning. Malignant melanoma, unlike the skin cancers discussed in chapter 7, can metastasize if not detected and treated early; for this reason, it is a potentially life-threatening form of cancer and should never be viewed as "just a little skin cancer."

Types of Melanoma

Many doctors divide malignant melanoma into four classifications: superficial spreading melanoma, nodular melanoma, lentigo maligna melanoma, and acral lentiginous melanoma. However, some authorities now consider these all to be variants of the same basic melanoma.

Superficial spreading melanoma is the commonest type, constituting 60 to 70 percent of melanomas in both men and women. It is an irregular brown, black, or bluish black growth, sometimes inflamed, with a tendency to ulcerate and bleed. Uncommonly, it may start from a preexisting growth, but more usually it appears as a new growth. If ignored or unrecognized, it may either metastasize or develop into a nodular melanoma (which may itself metastasize).

Nodular melanoma tends to be very fast-growing. It can arise on skin that had appeared normal or in a preexisting mole; it frequently ulcerates. Because it has a rich blood supply, it may resemble a blood blister.

Lentigo maligna melanoma (sometimes called *Hutchinson's melanotic freckle*) often arises on the face or some other sun-exposed area, often in older people. It is usually dull brown or black, with a very irregular lateral margin. It may remain in place (in which case the correct term for it is *lentigo maligna*) for years without metastasizing or invading neighborhood tissues. The appearance of raised nodules within it signals that it has begun to invade the dermis; at this stage, it is termed *lentigo maligna melanoma*. Although it can metastasize to the lymph glands, this form of melanoma is less likely to do so than either superficial spreading melanoma or nodular melanoma.

Acral lentiginous melanoma most often arises on the sole of the foot and sometimes occurs on the palm of the hand. It has a raised dark area, surrounded by a lighter area that may extend several centimeters around the raised area. A variety of this type of melanoma, called *periungual melanoma*, often arises in the region of the nail bed of hands or toes; it can easily be mistaken for warts or ingrowing toenails.

Melanomas can arise anywhere on the skin, under nails, and in hidden areas such as the genitals, the rectum, and membranes of the nervous system and the respiratory tract. Some melanomas arise in the eye, as will be discussed later in this chapter.

What Causes Malignant Melanoma?

Like other skin cancers, melanoma seems chiefly to be caused by exposure to ultraviolet radiation. Numerous studies indicate that, whether this UVR is obtained from sunlight or from artificial sources such as tanning salons, exposure increases a person's risk of developing melanoma later. Unlike other skin cancers, which usually develop from a lifetime of cumulative exposure, melanoma tends to be more common in Caucasians who have experienced intermittent and intense exposures—often in the form of a history of searing sunburns in childhood or adolescence. Research indicates that people who vacation in the sun, thus incurring a series of isolated bouts of sunburn, are more likely to develop malignant melanoma than those who actually work in the sun.

You have probably noticed that moles often run in families. Melanoma is linked to different types of moles—congenital (those present from birth or early childhood), acquired (those that develop later), or dysplastic (those that are unusual or atypical). Melanoma can develop even in people who have avoided the sun, especially if they have moles.

Other possible causes currently being investigated are immune system deficiencies, tumor-causing viruses, and chemical carcinogens. As discussed in chapter 2, exposure to ultraviolet radiation can bring about changes in the immune system. Moreover, the effects of UVR can be cumulative; and although it has not been established how exposing the skin at one site changes the immune response at a distant site, this effect has been demonstrated to occur. Margaret L. Kripke, professor and head of the Department of Immunology at the University of Texas's M. D. Anderson Cancer Center in Houston, says, "It is possible that local effects of ultraviolet radiation on immune cells in the skin might also play a role in the growth and spread of melanoma cells."

Types of Moles

Moles serve no function but in themselves are not dangerous; indeed, most of us have a number of these small colored spots, which are sometimes characterized as freckles or birthmarks. The average person's body has about twenty-five moles by adulthood. Some of these spots are present at birth, but most develop through life.

Unlike freckles, which lie flat on the skin, moles are elevated. The scientific name for a mole is *nevus*. Moles are usually brown, but they can range in color from pink to very dark brown because they contain cells similar to melanocytes, the pigment-producing cells found in the basal layer of the skin.

Congenital Nevi

These moles are either seen at birth or develop by the time a baby is six months old; however, they may be so light as to be barely noticeable. About 1 percent of babies are born with them. Generally, these moles run in families, and one or both parents may carry the trait. In some families you can see three generations of a family, all with a number of moles. People with congenital nevi are now thought to be at a higher risk of developing melanoma in later life.

Congenital nevi may never become troublesome, but some do develop into melanoma. Arthur Rhodes, MD, chief of the Division of Dermatology of the Children's Hospital in Boston, suggests that, if a pigmented mark is present on your child at birth, you should consult your physician. "Not all pigmented marks are moles," he says. "Congenital moles usually elevate the skin surface at least a bit when viewed from the side using a flashlight in a darkened room." Some flat brown marks may be café-au-lait spots, which are present in 1 out of every 100 white babies and 12 out of every 100 black babies. Mongolian spots may also appear. These are blue-gray and most often appear on the buttocks or back; they usually disappear by age twelve. Your child's pediatrician should be able to differentiate among these various marks.

Congenital nevi have been subdivided into three groups, according to their size in the person's infancy: small (less than 1.4 cm in diameter), medium (1.5 to 20 cm in diameter), or large (greater than 20 cm in diameter). Naturally these nevi will occupy different amounts of the body surface as the child grows.

Some physicians believe that medium and large moles should be removed, because of the high risk of developing melanoma in a large congenital nevi. If the mole looks normal, the physican may simply watch it carefully and consider removing it later in an office procedure. Many dermatologists photograph the moles to aid in maintaining careful observation of them over a period of time. Medium and large moles should be examined by the patient at home for any changes and every six to twelve months by a physician. If any changes develop in small or medium congenital nevi, the doctor will probably suggest either that it be removed or that a biopsy of it be performed. People with large congenital nevi have a 5 to 20 percent lifetime risk of developing melanoma, and for that reason some dermatologists prefer to remove them if doing so would not be cosmetically undesirable.

Anyone with nevi should watch out for and report the following danger signs:

* Changes in color (lightening or darkening)
* Changes in surface (a bump, a sore, or bleeding)
* Change in size (enlargement greater than can be explained by normal body growth)
* Pain or itching that lasts more than a few days.

These changes do not necessarily indicate cancer. But if cancer has developed, early detection and treatment are essential. Since people with congenital nevi are at a higher risk of developing melanoma than the general population, they should be especially careful to protect themselves against ultraviolet radiation.

Acquired Normal Moles

Some moles develop during the first thirty years of life, and these are termed *normal moles*. Most of them stay that way, but melanoma can develop in a normal mole. Thus, if one changes it should be seen by a dermatologist to assess whether the change signifies anything abnormal. Ordinary moles usually have the following characteristics:

* *Shape*: Round or oval; symmetrical with sharp, well-defined borders between the mole and the surrounding skin; may be flat, bumpy, or elevated
* *Color*: Uniformly tan, brown, or skin color; most look like others on the body
* *Size*: Usually less than 5 or 6 mm in diameter (slightly smaller than a pencil eraser)
* *Number*: In adults, usually ten to forty, generally scattered over the body
* *Location*: Concentrated on sun-exposed areas above the waist, such as the face, trunk, arms, and legs; seldom found on scalp, female breasts, or buttocks
* *Onset*: Usually appear during early childhood through mid-twenties; seldom after age thirty-five

Dysplastic Nevi

Some unusual moles are known as *dysplastic nevi*. The word *dysplastic* means abnormally developing. Such moles may develop at any time, but they are most likely to appear in adulthood. These moles are important to diagnose because studies indicate that people who have them are born with a tendency to develop malignant melanocytes. About 8 percent of Caucasians have dysplastic moles. The dysplastic mole itself may become malignant, or another mole or lesion may appear that is malignant.

It is possible (and indeed quite likely) for a person to have a combination of normal moles and dysplastic nevi. The latter may appear on both sun-exposed and sun-protected areas. Considerable evidence suggests that dysplastic nevi are related to sun exposure early in life, and that they tend to be larger in diameter and more numerous in sun-exposed areas than in sun-protected ones. Furthermore, research has substantiated that people with dysplastic nevi have cells that may be more likely to change when exposed to ultraviolet radiation than are normal cells. Studies also indicate that people with dysplastic nevi tend to be more susceptible to sunburn than people without these moles.

The tendency to develop dysplastic nevi may be inherited, or such nevi may simply develop randomly without any known family tendency to form them. Where dysplastic nevi exist in two or more family members, the condition is sometimes called *dysplastic nevus syndrome*. In families in which one or more members have developed melanoma, the risk of other members' developing the disease is extremely high.

If you have or suspect you have a dysplastic nevus, you should see your personal physician or a dermatologist. Dysplastic nevi look different from normal moles, but even an experienced dermatologist may have difficulty differentiating one from melanoma just by looking at it. Thus the physician may suggest a biopsy—the removal and microscopic examination of some or all of the suspected tissue.

If you have any question about whether your mole is a normal acquired one or a dysplastic one, err on the side of caution and see a doctor. Dysplastic nevi usually have the following characteristics:

* *Shape*: Irregular and often asymmetrical; the border may be irregular and seem to fade into surrounding skin
* *Surface*: Often pebbly or cobblestoned
* *Color*: Mixed and irregular, with speckles of tan, brown, dark brown, black, and red/pink within a single mole; moles may not look alike
* *Size*: Usually (but not necessarily) larger than a pencil eraser; some may be unusually large, even 8 mm or more in diameter
* *Number*: As many as 100, but there may only be a few
* *Location*: Usually found on the back, chest, abdomen, arms, and legs; also occur on areas not normally exposed such as scalp, buttocks, groin, or female breasts
* *Onset*: Many appear before age twenty-five, and appearance of new ones may continue through life; relatively stable once developed; new ones or growth in existing ones should be brought to a physician's attention

Dermatologists today are very careful to examine the skin of anyone who has dysplastic nevi, taking a family history and doing a biopsy on nevi that may look most suspiciously like melanoma. Allan C. Halpern, MD, Assistant Professor of Dermatology at the University of Pennsylvania, emphasizes the importance of diagnosing dysplastic nevi because people who get them have a high chance of developing melanoma by age fifty. He recommends frequent professional examinations (some specialists suggest follow-up examinations every 3 to 6 months) and what he describes as "aggressive observation." He also suggests taking photographs to maintain a record of any growths or changes. Thus, anything suspect can be removed; and if it is melanoma, it is caught when it is recently emerged and usually curable. Dr. Halpern, like all dermatologists, stresses that it is crucial for such individuals to avoid sun exposure.

Warning Signs of Melanoma

Malignant melanoma should be suspected if a new, pigmented mole develops in anyone over age forty; actually, any new growth or lesion, especially after adulthood, should be looked at by a dermatologist. Research shows that a number of people are not aware of the warning signs, do not realize that malignant melanoma can develop in a mole that has been present for a long time, or think that it can only begin in an existing one. The reality is that it can begin in either a preexisting mole or on "normal" skin.

Normal moles are usually:

* Smaller than a pencil eraser
* Of one shade or color, rather than a mixture

Normal moles should not:

* Itch
* Have ragged outlines
* Continue to grow in adult
* Be inflamed, bleed, ooze, or crust

A mole that deviates from the norm is not necessarily malignant, but it does warrant attention and should be checked out by a physician.

Melanoma may appear in a fingernail or toenail as a widening brownish or blackish band running up and down the nail. When such a band develops in a single nail, particularly in a person of middle age or older, a doctor's diagnosis should always be sought.

The American Cancer Society, the American Academy of Dermatology, and the Skin Cancer Foundation have devised a simple ABCD rule to help people remember some of the signs of melanoma:

A. ASYMMETRY: One half of the mole or growth does not match the other half.
B. BORDER IRREGULARITY: The edges are ragged, notched or blurred.
C. COLOR: The pigmentation is not uniform. Shades of tan, brown, and black may be present. Red, white, and blue may add to the mottled appearance.
D. DIAMETER: Any mole larger than 6 mm (the size of a pencil eraser) or exhibiting a sudden or continuing increase in size should be of special concern.

Here is a fuller description of the warning signs of malignant melanoma, as summarized in a brochure entitled *The Many Faces of Melanoma*, © by the Skin Cancer Foundation New York, NY (and reprinted here with permission):

* Change in size: especially sudden or continuous enlargement
* Change in color: especially multiple shades of tan, brown, dark brown, and black; the mixing of red, white, and blue; or the spreading of color from the edge into the surrounding skin
* Change in shape: especially the developing of an irregular, notched border that used to be regular
* Change in elevation: especially the raising of a part of a pigmented area that used to be flat or only slightly elevated
* Change in surface: especially scaliness, erosion, oozing, crusting, ulceration, or bleeding
* Change in surrounding skin: especially redness; swelling; or the developing of colored blemishes next to, but not a part of, the pigmented area
* Changes in sensation: especially itchiness, tenderness, or pain
* Change in consistency: especially softening or hardening

Who Is at Greatest Risk of Developing Malignant Melanoma?

For many years authorities thought that those at highest risk of developing malignant melanoma were people with red hair and freckles. True, the incidence is 7 to 10 times greater among people with fair skin, and it is 15 times more common in whites than in noncaucasians, but now it is known that a number of other variables affect a person's level of risk for this disease.

"Generally," says Allan Halpern, MD, of the University of Pennsylvania, "people at risk of developing malignant melanoma fall into one of two groups. The first is sun-sensitive Caucasians who blister easily from the sun, burn readily, tan poorly, or live close to the equator. The second group includes people who have a family history of malignant melanomas and have inherited the gene that places them at increased risk. They tend to develop a number of moles."

Dr. Halpern suggests that you be particularly on the lookout for changing moles that do not appear in obvious places like the forearms and face. Pigmented birthmarks are also at risk of turning into malignant melanoma.

People who have a number of dysplastic nevi are 22 to 30 times more likely to develop malignant melanoma than is the average person. Besides the fact that theses moles develop into melanoma, they are considered markers, identifying people who are also at an increased risk of developing malignant melanoma elsewhere on their bodies. Studies show that dysplastic nevi are larger and more prevalent in areas that have been exposed to the sun (especially during the person's first years of life) than in areas that have been protected. And a greater number of moles, in turn, increases the person's risk of eventually developing malignant melanoma.

Researchers have noted that the cells of individuals with dysplastic nevi show greater sensitivity and greater propensity to mutation (changes) from ultraviolet radiation than do normal cells. A person who has dysplastic nevi and a personal or family history of melanoma is thought to have almost a 100 percent risk of developing melanoma. But this circumstance should not unduly alarm you; remember that melanoma in its earliest stage is usually curable. Consequently, the Skin Cancer Foundation recommends that individuals in this very high-risk category personally check themselves and have regular checkups (total body skin examinations) at least once a year from a phsyician who specializes in skin diseases.

Approximately 15 out of every 100 melanomas of the skin develop in a congenital mole. Most congenital moles are small (less than 1.5 cm in diameter), but the lifetime risk of developing melanoma increases in individuals with large moles. It has been estimated that 5 out of every 100 people with congenital moles will develop melanoma by the time they reach age sixty. Melanoma occurs in young children only very rarely; but it may develop anytime after age twelve.

About 1 in 50 people who have been cured of a malignant melanoma are at extremely high risk of developing another melanoma within three years. This frequency is greatly increased (to 15 in 50) if the person has a relative with melanoma, because it tends to run in families.

Even if you conscientiously apply sunscreen or have little opportunity to be out in the sun now, you may be at risk. According to Arthur Sober, MD, dermatologist and melanoma specialist at Massachusetts General Hospital in Boston, "Even a single blistering sunburn in adolescence would double the risk of developing malignant melanoma later in life."

Some experts believe that if you have had a painful sunburn during the first 10 to 15 years of your life, your chances of developing malignant melanoma are tripled. Sidney Hurwitz, MD, clinical professor of pediatrics and dermatology at Yale University School of Medicine, states that, if all children used a sunscreen whenever they were out in the sun, from infancy until age eighteen, 81 percent of accumulated lifetime sun exposure would be eliminated. That would certainly lower the rate of melanoma for the next generation.

A number of studies have demonstrated that early intense exposure is responsible for the onset of melanoma. Careful investigation of the sun-exposure habits of patients who develop melanoma reveals that such patients frequently have, in addition to genetic risks (family history, moles, skin types, and so on) a history of a blistering sunburn in childhood or adolescence. These studies indicate that youngsters who were "poor tanners" (such as those with Type 1 or Type 2 skin) *and* had a blistering sunburn in childhood or adolescence were at greatest risk. But even "good tanners" were at serious risk if they spent long vacations in sunny areas during childhood, had a painful sunburn in childhood, and were often encouraged to be outdoors. Data show that individuals who are born in or who migrate to hot, sunny areas (southern United States, Australia, Israel) during childhood rather than during young adulthood are at very high risk. The time of arrival, rather than the length of time a person lived there, was a key risk variable. For instance, people who were born in western Australia or who arrived there before age ten had four times the risk of those who immigrated there after age fifteen; those who arrived before the age of ten also developed more moles on their arms than those who arrived later. Similar findings exist for Israel and New Zealand.

Children's personal schedules (no school in the summer; opportunities to be outdoors after school, on weekends, and even during recess at school) allow them to spend considerably more time outdoors than adults do, so it is easy to see how extensive their exposure to the sun can be. Unfortunately, this exposure can lead to melanoma twenty, thirty, or more years later.

Indoor workers have a higher risk for melanoma than outdoor workers, indicating that repeated, widely separated incidents of intense sun exposure in adulthood may be more likely to cause melanoma than daily, cumulative sun exposure. The reason is still undetermined, but among the various theories under consideration are several related to the effects of such bursts of exposure on the immune system.

The different types of melanoma are associated with different risks. Lentigo maligna melanoma usually arises on the sun-exposed skin of the elderly, strongly suggesting that years of sun exposure is a major cause. Superficial spreading melanoma, the most common type, places blondes, individuals with light or medium skin color, those with many freckles, and those who burn rather than tan or burn before tanning (Types 1 and 2 skin) at highest risk. People who have blonde, light brown, or red hair and light skin, but who can tan are at risk for nodular melanoma.

Although the incidence of malignant melanoma is considerably higher in Caucasians than in other racial groups, having dark brown or black skin is not a guarantee against melanoma. Black people, for example, may develop acral lentiginous melanoma, especially on the palms of the hand, the soles of the feet, under the nails, or in the mouth.

Four factors have emerged for placing people in the highest risk category of all: having spent more than two hours per day in the sun for ten to twenty years prior to diagnosis of melanoma; pursuing an indoor occupation in tandem with outdoor recreational habits; having light eye color; and evidencing poor tanning ability. Still, this list of special risk factors doesn't mean that the rest of the population is home free.

In some studies it has been shown that malignant melanomas most often do not develop from preexisting moles. Furthermore, those that do arise from moles are not always from dysplastic or congenital ones. But evidence indicates that, when melanomas do arise from moles, the moles usually were larger than 6 mm in diameter. This does not contradict the fact that people with dysplastic nevi are at great risk of developing the disease; rather it means that dysplastic nevi are markers for the development of melanoma *somewhere* on the body. For this reason, such individuals need to be especially careful to inspect their bodies for changes in the skin and to have frequent professional skin examinations.

Diagnosing Melanoma

If you have any of the warning signs of melanoma, see your personal physician or a dermatologist as soon as possible. Your personal physician will make sure that you are seen by a dermatologist, a general surgeon, or a plastic surgeon if there is any indication that you might have a melanoma. Remember, however, that even the most highly trained and experienced dermatologist cannot, just by looking, always determine whether a suspect lesion (new growth or existing mole) is a melanoma or not. Sometimes only a biopsy can provide the definitive answer; and if the answer is "melanoma," only a biopsy can determine the extent of the disease.

Frequently the dermatologist, general surgeon, or plastic surgeon will ask for another interpretation or reading of the slides (the sections of the growth prepared on slides and then reviewed by the pathologist) by one or two other pathologists. Often, the final and definitive report is "benign," meaning that the growth is totally harmless. Or you may learn that you have a "dysplastic nevus," which you should take as a warning signal that you may, at some future date, develop a melanoma. You know the rest by now: be especially vigilant for new growths and for changes in existing ones, and take precautions in the sun.

On the other hand, the laboratory report **may indicate** that the growth is a malignant melanoma. The report **will state** the extent of the malignancy, and your physician may want **you to** undergo some blood studies, X-rays, scans (computerized pictures of an organ or body part), or sonograms (computer pictures that use high-frequency ultrasound to examine the position, form, and function of anatomical structures), in order to determine the extent of the disease.

At one time, malignant melanoma was only diagnosed if the tumors bled, ulcerated, crusted, or grew large. Often the only reason a patient brought the condition to the doctor's attention was that it was unsightly. Usually these tumors had already progressed to a late stage, and even with surgery they were incurable. Fortunately, however, this is no longer so; and the change is due almost in its entirety to early diagnosis, after which effective treatment can be undertaken. Today, people with small growths that are not life-threatening are seeing their doctors and having the growths removed. And this, too, is increasing the cure rate.

In some unusual cases, metastatic melanoma may arise from a site other than the skin or eye; and in these cases a primary lesion is never found, despite intensive searching.

Predicting the Course of Melanoma

Although melanoma that is recognized and diagnosed early stands the best chance of being cured, a number of people delay seeking diagnosis and treatment. Why?

Some lesions may begin in an area that is not easily visible (the back, for instance), and as a result it is overlooked until it enlarges or is brought to a person's attention by someone else.

Many people who have little or no knowledge of the disease wait until the lesion is large, thick, and already invasive before consulting a physician about it. The American Cancer Society, the Skin Cancer Foundation, and hospitals and health groups throughout the country provide an important service in conducting screenings and in disseminating educational materials that help alert people to the signs of melanoma, in hopes of removing lack of knowledge from the roster of reasons for delaying diagnosis.

Still other people choose to ignore the warning signs, minimizing the seriousness because hiding their head in the sand reduces their fear and anxiety of cancer.

In a study conducted by Dr. Barrie Cassileth of the University of Pennsylvania Cancer Center in Philadelphia, it was found that patients waited an average of six months from the time they noticed changes in a mole until the time they decided those changes warranted professional examination. The study also established that people are more likely to be diagnosed early if they go to a dermatologist rather than to a phsyician for whom skin diseases are not a specialty. Experts cite this as a good reason to have regular examinations (at least when you recognize a warning sign or if you are in a high-risk category) conducted by a dermatologist. Anything suspect will then be removed (in whole or in part) and submitted for biopsy. The resulting reading of the extent of disease is closely linked to the prognosis (forecast of the disease's progress and probable outcome).

Melanomas observed in the earliest stage of development are thinner than those in later stages. When melanoma is diagnosed in its earliest and thinnest state, 99 percent of patients thus afflicted will survive for five years or more.

Still, no matter how alert you are to changes in your skin, it is possible that the diagnosis of melanoma may be made after it has begun to spread or invade beyond the site of its earliest stage.

The level (depth in skin) and thickness of melanoma, among other criteria, are referred to by pathologists as its *microstage*. Tumors with a low-risk microstage account for a growing number of the melanoma cases now seen by physicians. Such melanomas tend to be somewhat flat, but later they may develop a nodule.

Recent findings suggest that tumor volume, rather than just size, may be a critical factor in the prognosis of the melanoma. Reporting on a study of patients with malignant melanoma, Robert J. Friedman, MD, dermatologist at New York University School of Medicine, says that patients with tumors measuring less than 200 mm^3 had a nearly 90 percent five-year disease-free survival rate. In contrast, patients whose tumors measured more than 200 cubic millimeters had only a 10 percent survival rate for the same period. "Measurement of tumor volume [the portion within the dermis] may prove to be of significance in the prediction of survival rates," he told a roomful of physicians at the Forty-seventh Annual Meeting of the American Academy of Dermatology in late 1988. Dr. Friedman explained that measuring a tumor's volume may more accurately reflect the three-dimensional nature of tumors, in comparison with more common measurements that rely on a single dimension such as the level or thickness of the tumor. But until further studies are completed, the thickness of the original tumor will probably still be used as a major predictor of outcome.

Melanoma does its most severe damage (ultimately ending in death) by metastasizing (spreading) to the lungs, the liver, the neurological system, or other body structures and organs. How fast and where it will spread is not always predictable; there may be some association between where the melanoma initially appeared and where it goes next.

If metastasis has begun before diagnosis, surgery alone cannot cure the melanoma, but control of the disease is certainly possible. Treatment of melanoma is discussed in chapter 14.

Melanomas of the Eye and the Eye Area

Lentigo maligna, described earlier in this chapter, is a premalignant lesion that can develop on the eyelid. Malignant melanoma can occur on any portion of the skin, including the eyelids; however, melanoma accounts for less than 2 percent of all eyelid cancers. The growth may be tan or brown with irregular borders, and like other eyelid cancers discussed in chapter 6 this tumor requires surgical removal and (possibly) radiation for large lesions.

Melanoma of the eye is the most common cancer of that organ, but it is still rare. Some eye tissues contain pigment-producing cells in which melanoma can develop. As in the case of malignant melanoma of the skin, dark-skinned populations are at a lower risk than fair-skinned ones. The relationship between ultraviolet radiation and intraocular (within the eye) malignant melanoma has not been proved. However, one important study reported in the September 26, 1985, issue of the *New England Journal of Medicine* demonstrated that people who developed melanoma in the eye were more likely than the general population to have spent time outdoors in their gardens, to have sunbathed, or to have used artificial tanning devices. In addition, those who rarely wore hats, visors, or sunglasses while in the sun had a higher risk for developing the disease. All of this evidence certainly suggests that sunlight exposure is closely related to the development of intraocular malignant melanoma. Overall, the study's authors, who were associated with the National Cancer Institute and a number of prestigious medical centers, concluded that the risk factors involved in developing intraocular malignant melanoma are the same as those involved in developing it on the skin.

Melanomas can arise in the iris, in the ciliary body (which contains the muscles that control the shape of the lens), or in the choroid (the middle layer of tissue in the wall of the eyeball, consisting of blood vessels and dense pigment). Unfortunately, few signs or symptoms appear until the tumor reaches a relatively large size. Sometimes loss of vision, a sensation of floating spots, or protrusion of the eyeball may occur. It is also possible for tumor growth to cause secondary changes such as cataracts, glaucoma, or retinal detachment. The average age for developing this cancer is fifty, and there are no differences in rates of incidence between men and women. Intraocular melanoma is rarely associated with melanomas of the skin, since skin cancers do not commonly metastasize to the eye; however, it can spread from the eye to almost any organ of the body. Frequently it spreads to the liver, and sometimes melanoma of the eye is only diagnosed after it has already spread and appeared elsewhere.

Regular examinations by an eyecare specialist can help to diagnose this cancer before it spreads. Other diagnostic tests available are CT scans (the use of computers and X-rays to obtain a highly detailed image) and ultrasound, which can help to locate the tumor. Blood tests, radioactive scans, and other X-rays are used to determine whether the cancer has metastasized. Some tests may make use of a dye injected into a vein in the arm to highlight the blood vessels of the eye prior to taking an X-ray that may identify a tumor.

Treatments for intraocular and eyelid melanoma are discussed in chapter 12.

Malignant Melanoma and Pregnancy

Of the more than 27,000 Americans diagnosed with malignant melanoma in 1989, about 25 percent were under the age of thirty-nine. It is estimated that more women than men in this age group are so affected, which puts the spotlight on a growing problem: a number of women of childbearing age have had a history of melanoma. Hormones released during pregnancy stimulate melanocytes and promote the growth of pigmented lesions (it is common for normal birthmarks and moles to darken during pregnancy), but the precise relationship of these changes to the development of malignant melanoma has not been established.

If a woman develops melanoma during pregnancy, surgical removal of the lesion is usually performed; and if further treatment is indicated, it may be deferred until after the woman gives birth (if she is near term). Her progress will be monitored closely after pregnancy, and in all likelihood she will be told to delay subsequent pregnancy for at least two years and to avoid oral contraceptives.

Some physicians may even discourage women with a history of melanoma from becoming pregnant indefinitely. Such medical decisions are usually based on the extent of the disease at diagnosis. If the melanoma recurs within two years after initial diagnosis, the woman will probably be discouraged from ever becoming pregnant again.

Decisions about subsequent pregnancies should be made by a woman in consultation with her dermatologist and gynecologist. Some women may also wish to consult a medical oncologist—a physician who specializes in the medical aspects of cancer.

Early Detection Is Crucial

"If you catch a melanoma before it invades the dermis [the layer beneath the epidermis, where the mole is first noticeable], it is easily cured by outpatient surgery," says Dr. Allan Halpern. In this very early stage of malignant melanoma before invasion—called the *radial growth phase*—almost 100 percent of people will survive eight years if they have had the growth surgically removed. However, the deeper the melanoma grows into the skin, the more dangerous it becomes. If malignant melanoma spreads to the lymph glands, cure is extremely difficult to achieve; only 30 pecent of patients whose melanoma has reached this stage survive the disease. Sometimes micrometastisis occurs and cannot be detected at the time of diagnosis.

The heading of this subsection says it all. Early detection can result in surgical removal and cure. Later detection often involves combating a disease that is stubbornly resistant to treatment.

Reducing Risks of Malignant Melanoma

Stay out of the sun, avoid tanning salons, and see a dermatologist regularly if you have congenital moles, any unusual moles, or a large number of moles. Such preventive action may help you avoid developing melanoma at all, because any suspect lesion can be removed before it progresses to become malignant melanoma. If you have atypical moles, make sure that other family members are carefully checked too. And if someone in your family (a parent, grandparent, aunt, uncle, brother, sister, or child) has ever had melanoma, you should be examined for the presence of atypical moles or melanoma. If there is a tendency toward congenital moles in your family or if a child in your family has one, a thorough professional examination of your child should be conducted at puberty, when moles sometimes first assume the atypical appearance. Prevention and surveillance are the best defenses against malignant melanoma. Be sure to conduct self-examinations of your skin regularly, especially in hard-to-see areas, as outlined in chapter 7.

Remember that even individuals at high risk can reduce their life-threatening risk substantially. Melanoma that is recognized early and removed through simple in-office surgery can result in total cure.

Summary

Melanoma is a life-threatening illness that is becoming more and more common. It is closely linked to sun exposure (particularly searing sunburns in childhood or adolescence), to people with fair skin, and to congenital, acquired, normal, or atypical (dysplastic) moles. Some families tend to have congenital or acquired moles and to develop melanoma. Even people who have not had sun exposure can develop melanoma, and for this reason regular self-examination of skin and the reporting of any new growth or of changes in existing ones to a physician are essential practices for everyone to adopt.

The simple ABCD rule—asymmetry, border irregularity, color (nonuniform), and diameter (larger than a pencil eraser)—describes the major warning signs. A physician will remove and/or biopsy any suspect growths; and if it turns out to be melanoma in an early stage of development, it is usually easily curable. If the melanoma has begun to spread, treatment may still be successful.

Intraocular (within the eye) and eyelid malignant melanoma, while not very common, can pose risks to vision and to life. The causes of intraocular melanoma have not been fully determined, but they seem to be closely associated with those that cause skin melanoma. Regular examinations by an eyecare specialist and prompt reporting of any vision problems can afford a good chance for early detection and subsequent effective treatment.

As is the case with most cancers, early detection and early treatment are vital for curing all forms of malignant melanoma. Prevention is still better, and Part Two of this book focuses on this subject.

II

Protection from UVR and the Sun

9

Basic Care of Skin and Eyes

Protection from ultraviolet radiation—as well as from wind, cold, and heat—begins with sensible care of skin and eyes. Covering their bodies with clothes and sunscreen and wearing sunglasses constitute only part of the attention men, women, children, and adolescents should be paying to their skin and eyes.

Healthy skin begins with healthful living—plenty of rest and good food. Eat produce that is rich in vitamins A and C, dairy products fortified with vitamin D (especially important because you will be staying out of the sun and thus not getting your vitamin D from that source), and sufficient whole grains containing vitamin E, zinc, and selenium. Drink plenty of water or weak herbal tea, and minimize your intake of coffee, colas, and teas containing caffeine. And keep things on an even keel: be moderate with alcohol, stay away from the drug scene, and swear off smoking (which, aside from its other risks, constricts blood vessels in the face and causes premature aging).

Even the healthiest skin needs care, and this begins with clean skin. Although all skin, arms, legs, and other parts of the body need good care, our focus here will be on facial skin.

Cleansing the Skin

A suntan is no longer in fashion, according to the leading model agencies and fashion magazines, so people whose appearance is essential to their livelihood protect their skin year-round and take good care of it.

How do these men and women do this? The same way dermatologists recommend that you take care of your skin: twice a day, wash your face. Start the process by pulling your hair back. Then wash you hands well so that you don't add dirt and bacteria to your face, offsetting the good you achieve by cleaning it. Then lightly spread cold cream or cleansing cream all over your face and neck. You may prefer to use cleansing cream because it is thinner and lighter than cold cream, but the results are the same. With a good-quality tissue, gently remove the cream (and plenty of dirt) from your face and neck.

Now you're ready to wash your face. The old-fashioned method was to scrub your face with any kind of soap, and then rinse until it was squeaky clean. That may get your skin clean, but it certainly won't do anything to help keep it in prime condition. Use a mild soap that won't dry out the skin. Select it by its emollient qualities—that is, its ability to soften the skin. Among the popular-priced brands, Dove, Lux, and Camay are good; some dermatologists recommend more expensive alternatives such as Clinique or the transparent Neutragena.

Fruit, vegetable, and herbal soaps may be fun to use for the shower or bath, but they do nothing beneficial for your skin. Deodorant soaps may be fine for the shower, but they are far too drying for the face and can cause irritation and secondary yeast infections. Soaps described as "medicated" often have ingredients that by themselves are helpful for certain conditions but have not been proved to be effective when combined with the cleansing ingredients in soap. Moreover, they can irritate the skin.

After you have chosen your soap, you are ready. Work some of the soap into your wet hands, and then wash your face and neck well. Rinse with warm water until all the soap is removed. Then gently and carefully pat—don't rub—your face almost dry, and apply a good moisturizer, as described later.

At least once a week, you should exfoliate. Exfoliation is essentially a good scrubbing that removes the dead skin flakes that form daily on your epidermis as the skin regenerates. This procedure helps to rid your face of the dull, dry, and older-looking cells. The underlying skin of any age will look fresher and smoother, and the moisturizer will work better. Exfoliation is especially good for maturing skin, because it helps speed up the process of skin turnover, which has normally begun to slow down. Several companies make exfoliaters (sometimes called *scrubbers* or something similar), packaged in a jar or tube. These products have a grainy texture and are excellent for their purpose.

But don't overdo things. Dr. Albert Lefkovits, a clinical professor of dermatology at the Mount Sinai School of Medicine in New York and a member of the medical council of the Skin Cancer Foundation, warns patients against too much cleansing and exfoliation because it is easy to remove too much of the skin's natural barrier, drying out and irritating the skin. He also warns against too vigorous a use of synthetic or natural sponges that are designed to remove the top layers of the skin.

When men shave, they exfoliate that portion of their face; consequently, the extra use of the scrubbing products and the technique just described isn't as important for them as it is for women, but it's still a good idea! Everyone—men and women—should use a skin freshener (sometimes called a *toner* or *astringent*) daily. Just about every cosmetic and grooming company makes one; but if you're budget-conscious, you'll be interested to know that plain witch hazel works quite well. People with dry skin should use a freshener with low or no alcohol content. Fresheners complete the job of removing leftover cream, dirt, or makeup, and they close and firm skin pores.

This cleansing routine will leave your face feeling soft and moist, but it won't stay that way unless you hold in the moisture, which you can accomplish by using a moisturizer.

Moisturizing the Skin

Many people suppose that a moisturizer adds moisture to the skin, but that's not its purpose at all. When placed on a slightly damp skin, most moisturizers trap and hold the moisture that is already there; those that contain glycerin can attract additional moisture from the air to the skin. A moisturizer may be packaged in a tube, a jar, or a bottle. Lubricants, creams, skin softeners, vanishing creams, and emollients are often simply moisturizers by another name. Just be sure not to use one that is so thick that it clogs the pores. And if you have oily skin or a tendency toward acne, buy one that is advertised as noncomedogenic (indicating that it allows pores to breathe freely).

You may have heard that animal fats are good moisturizers. That's true, which is why you have probably seen advertisements for various fancy products that include fats from mink and turtles. But lanolin, a product of the oil glands of sheep, works just as well. However, Dr. Lefkovits says that lanolin can cause acne and allergic skin rashes, although products derived from it usually do not cause problems. My mother used to rub it on my face before I went out to play in the snow, and it certainly protected me from windburn, but if I used it at night it stained my pillow case. Still, it's an economical moisturizer to use when you are spending the day or a long evening at home, just reading or doing some chores.

Mineral oils, baby oil, and petrolatum or petroleum jelly are used as a base for many moisturizers. Vitamin E has often been proclaimed as therapeutic for aging skin, but its effectiveness for this purpose has not been proved. Dr. Lefkovits warns against opening vitamin E capsules and spreading the liquid on your face, since you may discover that you have a serious allergy to it. If you have a history of skin allergies, you should look carefully at the list of cosmetic ingredients on the packages of various products: vitamin E is often lisetd as *tocopherol acetate*.

How do you decide which moisturizer to use? A number of them feel wonderful on the skin, and the most expensive ones may feel especially good, but these are unlikely to offer you any more benefits than a simple moisturizer such as petroleum jelly. The FDA does not permit any product sold as a cosmetic to penetrate any deeper than to the upper layers of the dermis, so there is nothing that any of these products can do to encourage cell renewal, despite what some misleading ads may insinuate. And they absolutely cannot be absorbed and incorporated into the genetic material. (Prescription drugs are another story; we'll be discussing the remarkable Retin-A® in Part Three.)

Products that contain collagen are useful because they successfully hold in moisture, but collagen molecules are too thick to be absorbed into the skin, so store-bought collagen can't replace the natural collagen that has been worn away by age and sun exposure. Still, it can give you a younger appearance—at least for a few hours. That's because a number of cosmetics temporarily puff out the skin, making lines seem to diminish.

Find a moisturizer that you like because of its consistency, texture, fragrance (or lack of it), price, or availability. The one you use under makeup may be less protective than the thicker, greasier one you may prefer when you're not on public view. A number of moisturizers, as we will discuss in chapter 10, contain a sun protection factor (SPF) of 15 or more. Use the moisturizer(s) you decide upon every time you wash or wet your face, and before you go out; if you use makeup, always apply the moisturizer under it.

Extreme temperatures dry out your skin, so use it with even more frequency if you are going out in the cold or staying indoors in an overheated house. Air conditioning can deprive a house or office of moisture, so in that environment you may find you need to apply moisturizer during the day. Air pressure dries the skin, too; before you fly, be sure to apply an extra amount of moisturizer, and take some along on the plane to reapply during a long flight.

Apply moisturizer every night by spreading it all over your face and neck, smoothing it on gently with a light hand. Add an extra amount around your eyes. Try a moisturizer formulated for the eyes only; generally they are composed of lanolin, petrolatum, and other ingredients in a form that is not excessively greasy and is unlikely to irritate sensitive tissue. Your lips need greater protection than usual in cold weather and in the sun. A protective pomade or lipstick with a high sun protection factor will shield your lips from the elements.

When you shop for a moisturizer or any other product, take a good look at the ingredients before buying. As with prepared foods, the ingredients are listed in descending order on the basis of amount used. You will see that many such products contain petrolatum and lanolin, in addition to other ingredients. A *Consumer's Dictionary of Cosmetic Ingredients* (Revised Edition) by Ruth Winter (New York: Crown, 1989) is a good reference book to own.

Shaving

Some people assert that men's skin remains more youthful than women's because, when they shave, they also exfoliate. Despite protestations that they hate having to shave daily, most men like the way they look, feel, and smell after a shave.

To achieve a close, nondamaging shave, you should first soften the beard with warm water. Avoid using hot water, which can inflame the skin. To get a good lather, use shaving soap, lathering shaving cream, brushless shaving cream, or (most popular) shaving cream in a pump-style can. Lanolin and other lubricants are often built right into these products, along with pleasant scents such as lemon-lime, menthol, or a fragrance associated with a particular grooming line. These foams, consisting mostly of soap bubbles and air, hold moisture to the beard and soften and lift the hairs. Most are economical enough that you can use them generously. When *Consumer Reports* published a study some years ago on aerosol shaving creams, it reported that most of the panelists liked whichever one they tried. But be careful. Lime and certain other scents contain oil of bergamot, which is a photosensitizer; if you apply this to your skin and go out in the sun, you may get brown spots. In addition, avoid shaving creams that contain benzocaine, which can cause an allergic reaction.

Do not economize on your razor blades. They're relatively inexpensive, and a good stainless-steel blade coated with plastic will feel comfortable as it sails along your face. Six or seven shaves is the most you should try to get from one blade. Be careful not to stretch your skin when you shave; a light touch with long, even strokes along the grain keeps you from developing ingrown hairs. Have a styptic pencil handy in case you get a cut or nick.

Even if it's only for occasional use, an electric shaver is a good addition to a man's grooming essentials. You needn't choose between a traditional razor and an electric shaver: alternate as you wish.

After shaving—either with a razor or with an electric shaver—you may use cool water or a mild after-shave lotion to tighten your pores and smooth your skin. Most of these lotions consist of alcohol, water, glycerin, menthol, and fragrance. If you find alcohol irritating to your skin, choose a lotion that includes little or no alcohol.

Talcum powder, which many men use after shaving, accomplishes little besides spreading a thin white coating over the face and bathroom. But applying a mild moisturizer after shaving may be useful.

Types of Skin

In chapter 2 we discussed skin types in terms of fairness or darkness and in relation to their reaction to the sun. Here we will discuss skin types according to the categories oily, dry, normal, or combination skin. Each of these types of skin requires a different approach. It is useful to know your type before buying any products or embarking on a skin care routine.

Oily skin

People with oily skin usually have the following characteristics:

Enlarged pores
A tendency to have breakouts, acne, or blackheads
A shiny nose

If you have oily skin, you should keep your skin especially clean; but too vigorous scrubbing can have the paradoxical effect of irritating your skin and thereupon stimulating production of the oil glands, rather than ridding your face of the oil. Follow the same cleansing program described earlier, but buy products that have been formulated for oily skin. Don't be overzealous, or the skin may become too dry. In areas of skin that are oiliest and most vulnerable to breakouts or acne, use an astringent or toner that has a high alcohol content. You can use a moisturizer that is oil-free and specially formulated for oily skin. Women with oily skin should buy water-based (never oil-based) makeup.

Does diet trigger skin breakouts or acne? According to Dr. Lefkovits, "Foods containing iodine may aggravate acne. Therefore, avoid iodized salt, shellfish, and vegetables such as kale, kelp, seaweed, escarole, collard greens, and spinach."

If you find that stress plays havoc with your skin, you're not alone.

A number of people with oily skin say that their skin breaks out before final exams, job interviews, or dinner at the boss's home! Most dermatologists will tell you that this is not at all unusual.

There is a distinct advantage to having oily skin: people who have it are less likely to develop premature aging lines than are people who have dry skin (especially if they protect themselves from the sun). In time, though, even the oiliest skin is likely to become drier.

Dry Skin

People with dry skin usually have the following characteristics:

Almost invisible pores
A tendency to itch, flake, and get chapped
A tendency to develop tiny, premature wrinkle lines around the mouth or eyes

If you have dry skin, wash your face with soaps that moisturize, and apply astringents that contain little or no alcohol. Transparent soaps are good for sensitive skin, but since the added alcohol they contain draws water into the air, they can leave skin dry; therefore, it is particularly important to use a moisturizer promptly afterward. Hydration is essential for people with dry skin: a moisturizer helps lock in natural moisture, avoiding evaporation. Lips may need special protection, especially if they chap easily. In the winter, when your home or office is heated, use a humidifier or put a pan of water on the radiator.

Combination Skin

People with normal or combination skin usually have the following characteristics:

A supple, flexible, smooth texture
Essentially trouble-free skin

Even people who have this kind of skin (the majority of us) will have areas that may be dry one day and oily another. Some areas of the skin (such as the forehead and the eyes) may be dry, and other parts (such as the nose) may be oily. It is best to use skin care products labeled for normal skin, but it is also sensible to have available some products for dry and oily skin for use as needed.

Cosmetics and Makeup

Caring for your skin and protecting it from ultraviolet radiation will keep it healthy and attractive. But to enhance their appearance, most women choose to apply some makeup.

Most men don't wear makeup, but some do wear concealers or bronzers. A concealer does just what you would expect: it conceals blemishes. Bronzers (discussed in chapter 3) have been popular for years, but as more people realize that it is wiser to stay out of the sun, the bronzed look is becoming less popular.

No woman needs to maintain a huge collection of makeup. A complete supply might consist of the following:

A few different lipstick colors
One or two foundations (a darker or heavier one for evenings)
One light under-makeup moisturizer
One blusher and/or cream rouge
A concealer
A box of translucent powder
Three or four different eye shadows (although some makeup ex-
   perts believe that one is enough)
One eyeliner crayon
One brow colorer (powder or crayon)
One mascara

Optional items might include the following:

Lip glosses
Contour blushes
Lip-liner pencils
Eyeshadow sealer

The proper tools are necessary, too. You will need the following:

Some good quality sable brushes (the ones that come with makeup
   are not usually very good) for eyeshadow, powder, and blusher
A lip color brush
Disposable cotton swabs
Cotton (not synthetic) balls or squares

People can become allergic to the ingredients in a product at any time, even if they have been using it for years. If you suspect that you have developed a sensitivity to a product, and the problem doesn't clear up after you cease to use it, or if the reaction is severe, see a dermatologist. A number of companies describe their products as "hypoallergenic," but most types of makeup and cosmetics are formulated to promote as few allergic reactions as possible. Many people are bothered by fragrance and are happier using scentless products.

Care of the Eyes

When my husband and I gave his grandson a tool kit for his seventh birthday, he was thrilled. He said, "Everything I need is here."

His mother, Jacquelin Lustgarten, MD, smiled and said, "There's one thing missing. You know what it is?"

"My protective goggles," the boy answered.

She has trained her sons well. Sunscreens and sunglasses in the sun and eye protection whenever it is indicated are a normal part of their routine. Dr. Lustgarten is an opthalmologist, meaning that she is educated, trained, and licensed to provide complete eye care—medical, surgical, and optical—so she knows all the potential risks.

By and large, says Dr. Lustgarten, you don't have to do much to keep your eyes healthy and working at their best. Getting enough sleep, keeping away from harsh chemicals, and wearing protective goggles when your eyes are at risk of injury or of getting something (referred to as *foreign bodies*) in them are all the basic care you usually need. And Dr. Lustgarten adds, "People need periodic eye examinations at all ages."

Eye diseases can start at any time during life, and many do not cause symptoms until the disease has done damage. Since most blindness is preventable if diagnosed and treated early, regular examinations are important.

When Should Eyes First Be Checked?

It is best not to wait until problems arise before having your eyes checked. The American Academy of Ophthalmology and the American Academy of Pediatrics recommend that children's vision be screened regularly, starting at birth by the pediatrician or family physician. If any problems or abnormalities are noted at any time, the doctor will refer the child to an ophthalmologist. Some schools and school systems provide annual vision screening for all children. During the young adult and adult years, individuals at high risk of having eye problems (anyone with diabetes, hypertension, or a family history of glaucoma, cataracts, strabismus, retinal detachment, or some other hereditary or familial eye condition), as well as those taking medications that might affect the eyes, should be checked annually by an eyecare specialist. Others can be checked every two to five years.

The Eye Examination

An eye examination includes both a medical examination and a vision examination. You will be asked questions about your general health, your family's general medical and eye health history, any medications you are taking, and whether you are aware of any particular problems at this time. Then your vision will be tested with and without glasses.

Contact Lenses and Eyeglasses

Various abnormalities of vision still fall within the normal range of vision, even though all images may not be sharp. Such visual difficulties can be corrected with eyeglasses or contact lenses. Generally, the choice is up to you.

Protecting the Eyes

Everyone—children and adults alike—should take certain precautions to protect their eyes. Whether you need corrective lenses or not, you should wear polycarbonate goggles when playing sports (especially soccer, racquetball, and other ball games). Active youngsters should wear polycarbonate glasses at all times. Ordinary glasses may be more dangerous than no glasses at all; and those with what are called "shatterproof plastic" lenses are not sufficient. Be sure to wear protective goggles when you do any work that can produce wood, metal, or glass fragments or slivers; these can penetrate the eye. Always wear protective goggles when you work with chemicals, since chemical burns can lead to temporary or permanent loss of vision. As we discussed in chapter 3, never use any artificial tanning device without first donning totally opaque goggles.

Report any changes in vision (especially those of sudden onset) and any instances of pain or discoloration around the eyes to your physician or eyecare professional.

Caring for your eyes is more than just a matter of common sense; it is essential to ensuring continued trouble-free vision. In the next chapter we will discuss protecting your eyes from the sun.

Summary

Even the healthiest skin and eyes need basic care. Keeping skin clean and well moisturized and using products, tools, and cosmetics that are appropriate to skin type will help keep your skin in optimum condition.

Eyes too require care. Scheduling regular eyecare examinations and taking safety precautions against injury to the eyes are important ways to ensure that your eyesight remains as strong as it can be.

10 *Protecting Your Skin from the Sun*

The sun feels great, doesn't it? But good as it may be for the spirit, it certainly is not good for the skin. So today's smart look is a paler one, indicating that you have the good sense to guard your health by protecting your skin from the sun. In this chapter, we will discuss how you can achieve this protection successfully with the least effort.

As you will remember from chapter 1, ultraviolet radiation is emitted from the sun in three different wavelengths: ultraviolet A (UV-A), ultraviolet B (UV-B), and ultraviolet C (UV-C). UV-C is toxic to human, plant, and animal life, but it is filtered out by the earth's atmosphere, so it doesn't reach Earth. UV-B rays are the short, burning ones that worry most people because they penetrate the top two regions of the skin and are responsible for red, burning, and immediate damage to the skin. UV-B rays are at their most intense between 10 A.M. and 2 P.M. (11 A.M. and 3 P.M. Daylight Savings Time).

UV-A rays are of lower intensity than UV-B, but they can penetrate the third region of the skin, the dermis. UV-A's potential for long-term damage is great—even though it may not appear to burn the skin—because it is present all day long, year-round, whether the sky is cloudy or sunny, and sometimes even through window glass. It is especially concentrated during the early morning and late afternoon, when the sun is at an oblique angle overhead. Most people think of UV-A as the tanning rays and of UV-B as the burning rays, but all ultraviolet radiation causes both premature aging of the skin and skin cancer.

Often, people concern themselves with immediate health or beauty effects and forget about long-term effects. Thus, more effort has been expended on protection from the burning rays of UV-B than on protection from the equally damaging UV-A. One way to accomplish this is with the newer sunscreens, used reliably and correctly.

Back in 1987, a study indicated that fewer than half of all Americans used sunscreen products at all, and most of those who did failed to use them properly. Others thought that if they stayed under a beach umbrella they would be protected, forgetting that sand reflects a considerable amount of ultraviolet radiation. This reflected sunlight jeopardizes areas of the skin not generally exposed to the sun, such as areas under the chin and nose, or even the bottoms of the feet.

Most people are surprised to learn that sunscreens have been around for a long time. A chemical sunscreen containing a mixture of benzyl salicylate and benzyl cinnamate was introduced in 1928. Then in the 1940s, a Miami Beach pharmacist concoted a product (probably to protect his own bald head), using cocoa butter; he marketed it as Coppertone Suntan Creme.

Today's sunscreens are far more sophisticated and offer protection not available years ago. Every dermatologist, the Skin Cancer Foundation, and the Food and Drug Administration recommend that you use one. Taking precautions in the sun should become automatic, like placing small children in the car seat and buckling the seat belts on everyone else, even for a short trip.

Once it becomes a habit, you hardly even think about it. For instance, I use sun protection every day from May through October in New York, even if I'm just dashing out to mail a manuscript from the local post office. My husband, who once was an airline pilot for Uncle Sam, went on sun protection "automatic pilot" after I began researching this book. His hair is thinning, so he protects both his face and head by wearing a cap with a visor. We have learned by experience that sometimes one of us runs into an acquaintance with whom we stand chatting on the corner, finally going for a bagel or muffin and a cup of coffee. Then we decide to "walk it off" resulting in more than a half-hour of unanticipated sun exposure just when UV-A is at its strongest.

Questions and Answers about Sunscreens

How do you decide which sunscreen to use? If you go to a drugstore, variety store, or the cosmetic counter of a department store, you can easily be overwhelmed by the array of products displayed. However, the following question-and-answer format should help you decide what is best for you.

What are sunscreens?
Unlike the once-popular "suntan lotions," which encouraged a tan, sunscreens are substances applied to the skin that either absorb or reflect the sun's rays in order to prevent UVR from reaching the skin.

Are there different types of sunscreens?

All sunscreens work by blocking—to various extents—the harmful rays of the sun from penetrating the layers of your skin. Most of them only block UV-B, but some also protect you from UV-A. Sunscreens can be grouped into two categories: chemical and physical.

The chemical screens contain absorbing chemicals that act as a filter, absorbing solar energy before it can penetrate the skin. The absorbed energy excites the sunscreen temporarily, but then as the chemical relaxes back to its original state it transforms that energy into something harmless such as heat. This process of energy conversion is continuously repeated. Chemical sunscreens are usually colorless or a light white color, and form an invisible film on the skin, without altering appearance or staining clothing. Examples of active chemical agents are PABA (para-aminobenzoic acid), PABA esters, benzophenones, cinnamates, salicylates, and anthranilates.

Physical screens are usually opaque and contain ingredients that do not absorb UVR, instead reflecting and scattering the rays away from the skin. Examples of physical screens are those that contain titanium dioxide and zinc oxide. Physical screens are manufactured in bright, neon colors, as well as in the traditional white.

Because physical screens stain clothes, have a gritty consistency, and are messy to use, most people choose to use them only for very vulnerable spots such as the lips, the nose, and the helix of the ear.

Some physical agents are available in skin-tone colors for use by people with particular vulnerability, such as those with vitiligo (see chapter 2).

Do sunscreens protectd against both UV-A and UV-B?

Physical sunscreens reflect both UV-A and UV-B, thus protecting against both kinds of rays. Until recently, most chemical screens only absorbed the burning UV-B rays. Because they blocked out these rays, they often gave users a false sense of security and thus could actually promote a tan. Sunburn didn't occur, so people remained in the sun for longer periods of time, allowing UV-A rays to be absorbed into the deeper layers of the skin, with resulting long-term skin damage. But now some sunscreens do absorb both UV-A and UV-B; look for labels that say so.

Known as *full-spectrum* sunscreen agents, dibenzoylmethanes can protect against the entire UV-A waveband. These agents have been available in Europe and Australia for some time but were only introduced into American products in the late 1980s. One of these compounds, Parsol 1789, has been found to block much more of the

UV-A rays than oxybenzone (which has been available for a longer period of time). Combined with other chemicals such as Padimate-O, it provides excellent protection.

A number of cosmetic companies manufacture opaque makeup that performs as both a physical and chemical sunblock, offering broad protection.

What is meant by SPF?

SPF (or sun protective factor) is the ratio of the amount of energy required to produce a minimal sunburn through a sunscreen product to the amount of energy required to produce the same minimal sunburn without any sunscreen protection. For example, if you usually get slightly sunburned after 20 minutes in the sun without any protection, when you use a sunscreen with an SPF of 15 you theoretically will get the same sunburn only after staying out in the sun for $20 \times 15 = 300$ minutes, or 5 hours. However, SPF and tanning can be affected by your skin type, by the formulation of the sunscreen, and by the intensity of UV exposure. For instance, if you get sunburned at the pool or lake in Maine in 20 minutes, you might be badly burned in only 10 minutes at a high altitude relatively near the equator in New Mexico.

The Skin Cancer Foundation recommends that everyone use a sunscreen with an SPF of 15 or more. Little is known about the effectiveness of sunscreens with higher SPFs, although they most likely last longer and offer more protection during shorter periods.

It is important to recognize that SPF refers only to UV-B (the shorter, burning UV rays). Since UV-A rays do not produce a visible burn, protection from UV-A is not measured by SPF; instead, it is rated according to the percentage of UV-A that is blocked out.

Has the FDA made a statement about sunscreens?

Yes. Back in 1978, the Food and Drug Administration issued proposed rules that "would establish conditions for the safety, effectiveness and labeling of over-the-counter drug products." Sunscreens are considered drugs in the United States because their use can affect the structure or function of the skin; thus, they fall under FDA jurisdiction. The FDA allows sunscreen manufacturers to print the following notice on their labels: "Liberal and regular use of sunscreen products may help reduce the chance of premature aging of the skin and skin cancer."

Every sunscreen seems to say—contains PABA or PABA-free. What is PABA?

PABA (para-aminobenzoic acid) is one of the earliest-developed sunscreen chemicals. It is not used much today, because it causes an adverse skin reaction in a number of people (especially on skin that has been sunburned or windburned, and in areas around the eyes) and it tends to stain clothing. PABA has been around since the 1920s and was extremely popular until the introduction of PABA esters. These esters are strong yet nonreactive with the skin and far less likely to cause irritation.

Sunscreens described as "PABA-free" usually contain PABA esters.

Can sunscreens cause skin sensitivity in some people?

Unfortunately, they can. This is perhaps the main reason that PABA has declined so much in popularity and use. A number of users suffer redness and itching about 24 hours after applying sunscreens that contain PABA. The allergy may be caused by the PABA ingredient itself or by the combination of sunscreen plus ultraviolet light, resulting in a photocontact dermatitis. It is possible to be allergic to one form of PABA and not to others.

According to Leonard Harber, MD, chairman of the dermatology department at Columbia-Presbyterian Medical Center, 4 out of 160 patients in a study conducted there suffered an allergic reaction from benzophenone, which absorbs both UV-A and UV-B. The reactions ranged from itchy rashes to blisters.

Allergies can sometimes arise from other ingredients in the sunscreen, such as fragrances, preservatives, or the base used in formulating the product. Switching to another brand can make a big difference.

Reactions are usually temporary, but they can easily be misunderstood by people who think that their allergy is to the sun; instead of changing sunscreens, these people may use more of it or may switch to a version of the same product that has a higher SPF. The greater concentration of chemicals in the product may simply increase the sensitivity.

Individuals who have a history of allergies—especially to hair dyes, sulfonamides, or procaine—or who are taking antihypertensive or diuretic drugs may be sensitive to PABA and PABA esters. Discuss your situation with your doctor before using sunscreens that contain these ingredients, or ask if it would be safe for you to do your own patch test. Apply the sunscreen to a small patch of skin (preferably on the underside of the forearm) and then cover the area with a small adhesive handage. Then after 24 hours, remove the bandage. If there is any redness or swelling of the covered area, don't use that sunscreen. But even if there is no reaction, expose the area to 15 minutes of sunlight and then wait another 24 hours. If a reaction appears the next day in the form of redness or swelling, your test is positive and you should avoid this product.

Cinnamates are used in a number of sunscreens. Some people who are allergic to them are also sensitive to cinnamon-flavored products such as mouthwashes, chewing gum, and toothpastes.

Some of the new broad-spectrum sunscreens can cause allergic reactions in some individuals—especially those who are sensitive to benzocane, sulfonamides, or PABA.

If you are unable to stay out of the sun, and can only tolerate chemical sunscreens with a low SPF, your druggist may be able to combine it with a titanium dioxide paste, to afford you a safe and nonallergenic sunblock.

Don't become unduly alarmed by this discussion, because the overwhelming majority of people have little or no sensitivity to sunscreens.

Are some sunscreens genuinely waterproof?

Yes, they are. The vehicle or base containing the UVR-absorbing chemical determines the sunscreen's effectiveness under various conditions, such as immersion in water. A sunscreen's ability to adhere to your skin while you are sunbathing, sweating, or swimming is called its *substantivity*.

Sunscreens that contain PABA esters such as Padimate-O are considered very substantive. Sunscreens that use an oil or cream base are more water-resistant than those that use an alcohol base.

If a sunscreen is labeled *waterproof,* it must maintain its rated SPF for 80 minutes in water. Sunscreens that are *water-resistant* are supposed to maintain their SPF for 40 minutes in water. Interestingly, some products actually have a higher SPF than is labeled on the product so that, even if some of it is washed away, the sunscreen will still offer the advertised protection.

Waterproof sunscreens are an excellent choice if you plan to be swimming or dodging ocean waves, and the water-resistant ones are good if you are active and anticipate perspiring.

After swimming in a chlorine-filled pool and drying yourself vigorously with a towel, don't expect your sunscreen to continue to be effective. Play it safe—even if you dry naturally—and reapply sunscreen.

Do sunscreens come in different formulas?

Most sunscreens are sold in bottles and tubes as lotions or creams. The clear lotions seem more like liquids; their advantage is that they're not greasy, so sand doesn't stick to the skin. Clear lotions usually have an alcohol base, and are especially good for people who have oily skin. Some people complain that they find it difficult to determine whether they have covered all of their skin when using a clear lotion.

Most cream formulas are not especially greasy; and although they go on creamy white, they disappear when rubbed in. It is easier with cream formulas to see if you have missed any spots.

Various under-makeup moisturizers have an SPF of 15. They offer a good way to protect your face, with or without makeup. If you are planning to be out in strong sun or for a long period of time, however, you will want to add additional sunscreen.

Sunscreens may be packaged in tubes (like ointments), in spray containers, in stick form, or in plastic bottles. Some are lightweight gels that absorb into the skin instantly. Individually wrapped sunscreen towelettes are perfect to put into your bag or pocket or to leave in your desk drawer for unexpected outings. Hair sprays often have an SPF built into them. This feature helps protect hair color from oxidizing, and it may give some protection to scalp, but a low-SPF hairspray will not sufficiently protect scalp if the hair itself doesn't provide a good barrier.

How do you choose a sunscreen?

Wisely, we hope. Don't just grab the first bottle or tube that you see on the counter. Think about how you will be using it. Will you just be wearing it while walking through the shopping area of your city, sightseeing on a vacation in a foreign city, or sitting quietly on your front porch reading the paper? If so, you will not need a sunscreen that is waterproof or water-resistant.

If the weather is hot, or if you plan to be running after the kids in the park, participating in any sports, or encountering some water, you will certainly want a water-resistant sunscreen. If you will be swimming, a waterproof sunscreen is essential.

The Skin Cancer Foundation recommends that everyone use a sunscreen with an SPF of 15 or more. Remember, a sunscreen with an SPF of 15 or more costs only pennies more than one with less protection. If you still feel you want a bit of a tan, start by using sunscreen with an SPF of 15 or more, and then later in the season use sunscreen with a lower number. A sensible tan like this shouldn't get you into any major health trouble; but remember, it certainly will accelerate skin aging. There is no way around this simply rule: tan now, pay later.

Is an expensive sunscreen better than a moderately priced one?
Better is a tricky word. Will an expensive sunscreen protect you more? No. Will it appeal to you more because of its texture, fragrance, packaging, or dispensing qualities. Perhaps. An SPF is an SPF, and whether you buy your sunscreen at a large discount chain store, or at a fancy cosmetics counter in a department or speciality store, you should be getting the same protection. Stay with a brand-name company, if you feel more confident about its products, and remember that good turnover assures you of a fresher product. Appendix I tells you how to receive a listing of sunscreens that are recommended by the Skin Cancer Foundation.

Is there a special way to apply sunscreens?
Naturally, you should follow directions on the bottle. But many manufacturers neglect to tell you how important it is to apply a sunscreen before going out in the sun. Experts say that it takes at least 30 minutes for a sunscreen to sink into the skin. Sunscreens with PABA should be applied 2 hours before exposure.

Sunscreen binds best to cool dry skin, and you'll miss far fewer spots if you remember this and use some common sense. Always put the sunscreen on before you put on your bathing suit or clothes. That way you won't miss areas of demarcation, where the clothes end and you begin! Be generous with sunscreen; and if you use a cream formula, leave a film that you can feel. Some oil-free screens are designed to disappear, so they will not leave a film. Apply the sunscreen over all exposed areas of your body, and consider using an additional thick dab of physical screen on "hot spots."

How much sunscreen should I use?
More than you probably think. The average adult wearing a bathing suit should plan to use ½ teaspoon on *each* of the following parts of the body: the face and neck; each arm and shoulder; the front and back of the torso; and each leg and top of the foot.

Most people are rather stingy with their sunscreen and don't use enough for proper coverage. It is better to use plenty of a lower-SPF sunscreen than not enough of a higher-SPF sunscreen.

How often does sunscreen need to be applied?
The Skin Cancer Foundation suggests that you apply sunscreen before every exposure to the sun and that you reapply it frequently and

liberally. They suggest doing this every two hours, as long as you stay in the sun, and reapplying it after swiming or perspiring heavily.

Just becaues an SPF seems to give you the protection you need for a few hours (according to the mathematical equation given earlier) does not mean that you are fully protected for that amount of time. Rather than playing the numbers game, use an SPF of 15 or more, and apply it frequently.

Is there a way to protect the head if you are bald or hair is thinning?

Bald-headed men must protect their head in the sun, since this skin is very vulnerable. Wearing a sunscreen and a cap while sitting in the sun is essential. But people with thinning hair face a difficult dilemma. Hairsprays with an SPF built into them are useful for people with thick hair, but the SPF is usually too low to provide protection for exposed parts of the scalp, so wearing a hat or cap is probably the only way to get complete protection. But most men prefer not to wear a bathing cap while they are swimming or to wear a hat when they are dressed in a business suit. A product made by Dermatone called Topcoat is a good solution. It is an aerosol (free of ozone-depleting chlorofluorocarbons) that sprays through thinning hair directly onto the scalp. It is waterproof and has an SPF of over 20. Undoubtedly other manufacturers will be introducing similar products in the future.

When should you use sunscreen?

You should use sunscreen whenever you are going to be exposed to sun for any period of time. If you are just going to spend lunch hour (when the sun is strongest in UV-B radiation) sitting in the park across the street from your office, you need protection. If you are going to the beach for the day, even if the weather report is for hazy, overcast weather, you need sunscreen, because UV-A comes right through those clouds.

Protect your hands, arms, and other exposed areas with sunscreen (or appropriate clothing) when you fish, jog, ski, or play golf, tennis, or other outdoor sports. Protect your lips with a balm that has maximum sunscreen; women can use a lipstick that offers protection. Any time you are out in midsummer or at high noon, are surrounded by sand or snow, or are in the tropics, use maximum protection.

You need sunscreen even when you are going to be sitting in the car, unless you are sure that you will be keeping the windows closed. I learned this quite graphically last summer. The air-conditioning in my car was giving me trouble, so I drove with the window open. My face was well protected because I apply a moisturizer with an SPF of 15 under any makeup or, more often, wear makeup that provides a total sunblock; but I hadn't bothered to protect my arms because I wasn't planning to be outside for more than a few minutes at a time. Within a week I had a "watch strap mark," indicating that the sun had gotten to me after all! Even if I had remembered to use a sunscreen on my hands and arms, if it weren't a broad-spectrum one that blocked out much of the UV-A as well as the UV-B, I would probably have tanned. Moreover, a car's side windows do not usually block out UV-A.

Many women use a good-quality broad-spectrum sunscreen as a moisturizer under makeup (allowing a half-hour for it to set before applying makeup) and also put some on their hands and arms to avoid acquiring age spots. Men should apply sunscreen after shaving each morning.

A surprising statistic tells us that 80 percent of sun exposure is incidental. Your skin absorbs those rays when you do errands, walk the dog, push the baby carriage or shopping cart, or simply walk to and from lunch. That adds up to a lot of cumulative exposure, and although you are not likely to get a sunburn from these errands, the damage is accruing in the third layer of your skin, the dermis. Eventually you will pay the penalty with prematurely sun-damaged and aged skin and perhaps with an increased risk of cancer.

Wouldn't an overall even tan offer some protection against sunburn?

It may offer you protection against the searing sunburn you would have gotten without the tan; that's precisely the selling point that tanning salons try to use. But the truth is that a tan is not healthful; instead, it is the recorded evidence of damage that the skin has suffered. A suntan offers no more protection than a sunscreen with a 2 or 3 SPF, which is minimal. Thus, even with a tan, damage will accumulate.

How long can you store sunscreen?

This is a tough question. First check the bottle to see if there is an expiration date on it. Some sunscreens require this, but others have ingredients that don't lose their potency, so there may be no date.

The FDA doesn't require an expiration date on most sunscreens because they are thought to be stable for at least three years, but many authorities say that one year is the longest you should keep a sunscreen. The oil can separate from the solids in some products, downgrading the SPF, and the SPF can also deteriorate from exposure to heat. A good idea is to mark the date you purchased the sunscreen, so you will know later how long you have had it. Avoid storing opened or closed sunscreens in warm places such as medicine cabinets in bathrooms. Try to buy the product at a store that has a high turnover; look at boxes and bottles and notice whether they seem free of dust and dents.

Children need sunscreens, too—don't they?
They certainly do, although sunscreen companies instruct you not to use these products on babies before the age of six months. Consult your pediatrician if some sun exposure seems unavoidable. Whenever possible, keep baby out of the sun altogether, as discussed in chapter 5. A little later we will discuss some additional ways of protecting babies from the sun.

By the age of one year, children should be using sunscreen. If you have any questions about starting to use it earlier or waiting longer, discuss these with the baby's doctor. You can purchase sunscreens that are clearly targeted for children, or you can buy any non-PABA milky lotion or cream. Avoid clear lotions, which may contain alcohol and can sting.

When applying a sunscreen, avoid covering the eyelids (kids love to rub their eyes), because the ingredients can irritate the eyes. Apply it generously to all uncovered areas; putting little dabs on the face and shoulders is not enough. Reapply the sunscreen frequently—every 60 to 90 minutes it not too often. Be sure to apply sunscreen under sheer fabrics such as thin T-shirts or light, lacy bathing suits, since the sun can penetrate thin wet fabrics.

If you screen out all the sun, will you develop a vitamin D deficiency?
Probably not, if you are eating a normal diet—particularly one that includes milk and milk products fortified with fat-soluble vitamin D. Foods rich in vitamin D are egg yolk, liver, tuna, salmon, and cod liver oil. Dark-skinned people in cold climates and people who habitually wear a total sunblock and clothing that doesn't permit any UVR to penetrate should, for added protection, take a high-potency multivitamin formula containing 400 IU of vitamin D. This will supply the United States required daily allowance (RDA). Vitamin D, sometimes called the "sunshine vitamin," is transformed by kidney action into a more potent form, in which it assumes the role of a hormone. It is secreted into the bloodstream, where it helps to control

the absorption of calcium from the digestive system, maintaining healthy bones. It is needed by adults, as well as by children. Bodies make their own vitamin D, but the energy from ultraviolet light helps to activate its production. Most experts say that about 15 minutes of exposure to sunlight two to three times a week by any area of the body is sufficient.

Individuals who don't go out at all (such as nursing-home residents) or who work a schedule that allows them little fresh air (except perhaps in a heavily polluted area) and who may not be getting enough fortified foods (this can include vegetarians who don't eat any meat by-products, including homogenized milk or eggs) require a vitamin D supplement.

But you should avoid megadoses. Excess vitamin D is stored in the liver, and a surplus of it can cause serious problems. From too much vitamin D, adults can develop deposits of calcium throughout their body, deafness, nausea, loss of appetite, kidney stones, fragile bones, high blood pressure, high blood cholesterol, or increased lead absorption.

Babies need vitamin D in order to avoid rickets. Doctors no longer advocate the old-fashioned "sun bath," because vitamin D is now added to formula; instead they tell you to keep the baby out of the sun. Nursing mothers are advised to give their babies a vitamin D supplement, frequently contained in a multivitamin preparation. This is particularly important in relatively cold climates, in the winter, and in severely polluted areas, when many babies are rarely taken outdoors. Use only the amount recommended by your pediatrician, because megadoses of vitamin D in infants are extremely harmful; risks associated with megadoses in infants include calcium deposits in the kidneys and an excess of calcium in the blood. As with so many good things—medication, vitamins, or even healthful food—more is not always better.

Should elderly people use sunscreens, too?

Absolutely. They don't want to develop skin cancer, and because their lifetime exposure to the sun began in the days before the dangers were recognized, their cumulative exposure is already great. Many older people have already had one or more skin cancers, so they must be extremely cautious.

Studies have indicated, however, that older people who use sunscreens with an SPF of 15 daily may have less than half the vitamin D level of those who don't use it. Rather than cutting down on SPF, take a multivitamin that includes vitamin D, or take an additional vitamin D supplement. Don't overdo it, though, or you risk incurring vitamin D toxicity. Very little sun exposure is needed to spur the skin to manufacture vitamin D—far less than the amount needed to cause sunburn or tanning. Solar radiation may also penetrate light clothing sufficiently to help manufacture the vitamin.

After years and years of sun exposure, is there any value in starting to use a sunscreen now?
Yes. It's not like closing the barn door after the cow gets out: it is never too late to begin protecting your skin from further assault. One exciting development is the news that dermatologists now believe that protection from the sun—either through use of a sunscreen or as a result of staying out of the sun altogether—may allow the skin to regenerate collagen and elastin, the tissues responsible for keeping skin smooth.

Is there legitimate concern that some ingredients in sunscreens pose a health risk?
In the spring of 1989, a report in the media stated that some sunscreens were potentially dangerous because certain ingredients may break down, producing a substance (known by the acronym NPA-BAO) belonging to a class of chemicals called nitrosamines that can be termed *carcinogenic* (cancer-causing). In response to concerns about the safety of sunscreens, the Skin Cancer Foundation issued a statement from Madhukar A. Pathak, a senior associate in dermatology at Harvard Medical School and chairman of the Photobiology Committee of the Skin Cancer Foundation, and Perry Rogers, MD, Associate Professor of Clinical Dermatology at the New York University School of Medicine and president of the Skin Cancer Foundation. These experts explained that the amount of NPABAO detected in certain sunscreens is quite small and that it is probably organized as a breakdown product of an uncontrolled chemical reaction of the sunscreen ingredient Padimate-O, which has been used for more than fifteen years. There is no known interrelationship between Padimate-O and skin cancer; and the FDA, which conducted tests of the sunscreens, emphasized that no testing has been done to determine whether the specific substance NPABAO is a cancer-causing agent and cautioned against extrapolation from the reported observations. Doctors Pathak and Robins stated, "Since NPABAO belongs to a class of chemicals known as nitrosamines, some of which have been shown to cause cancer in animals, we, as physicians and representatives of the Skin Cancer Foundation, are naturally anxious to know the immediate

as well as the long-term consequences of these hitherto unknown or uninvestigated compounds."

These experts believe that a long-term study of NPABAO is needed; but in the meantime, they concluded, "We feel it is important to assure the consumer that the sunscreen products produced by the leading American manufacturers are indeed superior in their photo-protective qualities. We strongly recommend that people continue to use sunscreens with a high sun protection factor (SPF 15 or higher) *with* or *without* Padimate-O." If you're worried about possible ill effects of this ingredient, choose a sunscreen that does not contain it.

Is there a way to know how much ultraviolet radiation is reaching us?

Unfortunately, such information is not readily accessible to most of us. But one company—Solar Light Co. of Philadelphia—has produced a weatherproof sunburn UV meter for continuous recording of ambient levels of sunburning ultraviolet radiation. This meter consists of an outside sensor cabled to an indoor data acquisition system; it provides information for meteorological records and for local radio stations to broadcast warnings.

Wouldn't it be wonderful if all weather reports included information about the amount of ultraviolet radiation likely to affect us? Then we would know whether we needed to pack sunscreen in our bag or briefcase along with (or instead of) our umbrella, and frequent updates would help us plan protection all day.

Why is it that some people just won't use sunscreen—even though they know better?

Good sense tells most of us to take precautions against aging skin and cancer, and the same good sense makes us wonder why some people refuse to heed warnings.

Psychologists at the University of California at Riverside wondered, too; so Howard S. Friedman and Barbara Kessling conducted a study, published in *Health Psychology* in 1987. For this study they interviewed sunbathing and nonsunbathing beachgoers about their health practices, kowledge about skin cancer, moods, and thoughts about the social rewards to be obtained through sunbathing. One finding was a partial confirmation of a stereotype of sunbathers as individuals who are relaxed but very concerned with their appearance. But another portrait also emerged: an action-oriented, risk-taking person who values the appearance (as opposed to the careful nurturing) of health and who associates with like-minded individuals. Sunbathers, Friedman and Kessling found, were far less concerned with actual health than with the appearance of health, and although many of them exercised and maintained the right weight they tended to be risk-takers as far as other health behaviors are concerned. As regards the dangers of UVR exposure, many professed ignorance; others just paid no attention to warnings.

Some people simply avoid listening to the odds or hear them but think that they won't be "unlucky." Perhaps that's why Las Vegas is full of people—some at the gaming tables, and others sitting around the pool, basking in the hot sun!

Other Ways to Protect the Skin

Sunscreens are an excellent way to protect your skin from the sun. Invisible, easy to use, and always available, sunscreens can afford you safety while enjoying the great outdoors anytime and anywhere.

For additional safety, or when frequent application of sunscreens is not desirable, you can adopt other ways to protect your skin.

Clothing

Whenever possible when sun exposure is inevitable, wear long-sleeved shirts and long pants made of lightweight but tightly woven fabrics. Hold an article of clothing up against the light. The less you can see through it, the more protection it will give you. Fibers that are sheer enough to see through seldom provide much protection; the sun simply goes through them. Tighter weaves—preferably dyed—allow less sun to penetrate to the skin. The darker the fabric is, the more light and heat it will absorb; and so on a hot day it may be quite uncomfortable.

In the Middle East, the most popular clothing color is white. When white clothes cover most of your body, they can absorb about 70 percent of the sun's radiation and reflect another 10 percent, thus keeping you cool. But thin white wet clothing, especially after you have been swimming or perspiring, permits UVR penetration. Remember this when you wear tennis whites before a strenuous match or plan to buy that beautiful white bathing suit.

Polyester fabrics present less of a barrier to UV-B than do cotton ones, although some specially woven semitransparent polyester fabrics may partially block the burning rays.

Experimental studies with fabrics precoated with UVR-absorbing chemicals show remarkable success. Dr. Madhukar A. Pathak is enthusiastic about a new chemical process capable of absorbing UV-A and UV-B that is bonded to the fabric, thus eliminating all UVR to skin. He feels that an important future protection lies in pretreating fabrics with these chemicals to produce clothes offering an SPF of 50, 60, or even 200. The protection lasts through 25 washings and even develops more UVR resistance. Essential for outdoor workers, such clothes would also be excellent for people who choose to spend leisure time outdoors. Look for them in your local stores or by mail order.

Hats

A hat with a wide brim or a baseball-type cap offers good protection for the head and forehead, and supplemental protection for the eyes. A visor alone can protect the forehead and eyes. For optimum protection—either because you will be out in the sun for hours on end (while fishing, perhaps) or because you are at particular high risk—a hat that offers more extensive coverage is useful.

Look for hats with large brims and flaps that can protect the face, ears, and neck. Find one that is light, durable, and made of cotton or a combination of cotton and polyester.

Head coverings like these are appropriate not only for outdoor enthusiasts, but for all outdoor workers, lifeguards, gas station attendants, and beach attendants. A retired businessman and golfer who has suffered from skin cancer himself and has marketed such a hat, James McCracken believes that employers should provide outdoor workers with a sun-protector hat. Citing illnesses resulting from hazardous work conditions, he poses a provocative question: "In ten to twenty years, will employers who do not provide or warn employees who work in the sun to use sunscreen, wear a hat, and take other precautions be sued by employees who get skin cancer?"

Umbrellas, Parasols, Awnings, and Such

Such items are useful indeed, but don't count on them for total protection. Staying under a beach umbrella or other covering outdoors only gives you partial protection, because the sun's rays scatter and can get to you even under an umbrella. Coverup clothing, sunscreen, and shade are all vital elements of your defense against the effects of the sun.

Windows and Glass

Most windows and glass screen out UV-B, and some of the newer ones block out some UV-A. If you are putting new windows into your home, look for those with low-E coatings; they block out a lot of the sun's ultraviolet rays and also keep furniture and fabrics from fading.

Glass generally does not serve as a complete barrier between you and ultraviolet radiation. So if your desk is right next to a window and you have been enjoying that beautiful sunlight and view, remember to put a broad-spectrum sunscreen on each day before going to work. However, as long as you don't sit right at the window "soaking in the sunshine," you probably won't need this protection unless you are going to be outdoors.

The windshield of your car, because of its slant, screens out a great deal of the sun's UV-A, but the side windows don't do a very good job of it. Therefore, if you are planning a long car ride, or if you spend a great deal of time each day in the car (even with the windows closed and the air-conditioning on) take precautions: use sunscreen and wear coverup clothes.

Protecting Babies and Children

Unless your pediatrician suggests otherwise, you should not apply sunscreen to babies under six months of age. But there are a number of ways of protecting babies and young children without keeping them indoors all summer (or year-round in the Sunbelt).

A number of excellent products are available to help shield babies from reflected sunlight. Some playpens come with their own canopy or shade; or separate canopies and shades can be purchased to attach to the playpen you already have. Baby hats with foreign-legion-style flaps offer more protection than do conventional hats. Washable shades attach by an elastic hem to carseats or infant carriers, for partial or complete shade; fiber mesh shades attach with velcro to standard carseats; and a number of shades are made to attach to carriages. Carshades that attach to car windows with suction cups work just the way home window shades do and will afford added protection to small children sitting in the backseat of the car.

Protective products of the types listed above are available in many stores. If you can't find them where you live, various mail-order companies often gather unique and useful products to list in their catalogs. One company committed to sun protection for small children is The Right Start Catalog in Westlake Village, California. Call them at 1-800-LITTLE-1 for a catalog or for more information.

Summary

Sunscreens are essential for protecting skin from the deleterious effects of the sun. Vastly improved in recent years, sunscreens generally fall into one of two categories: physical agents (for example, zinc oxide) or chemical agents (for example, PABA and PABA-free chemical compounds). Those with an SPF of 15 or more offer optimal protection when properly applied. Newer sunscreens protect against both UV-A and UV-B and are available in water-resistant and waterproof formulas. Even people who have a sensitivity to ingredients in one type of sunscreen can usually find a sunscreen that meets their needs.

Sunscreens today are generally safe and effective. They can and should be used by everyone, from young children to the elderly. Fears that vitamin D deficiencies will result from regular use of sunscreens are unfounded; a vitamin D supplement can be taken by those whose diets do not include enough of it.

Protective clothing and hats should be worn outdoors and the sun should be avoided when it is at its strongest.

11 *Protecting Your Eyes from the Sun*

The world certainly looks brighter on a sunny day; the grass and pavements glitter, and the skies are the bluest blue. Why dim it all with sunglasses?

As a matter of fact, there are several good reasons. Glare from the sun can give you a headache and make you squint (helping to set those fine lines and wrinkles), and large amounts of visible and invisible ultraviolet (both UV-A and UV-B) light can be harmful to the eyes. In addition, bright sunlight can damage the cornea, the lens, and the retina of your eye.

As we discussed in depth in chapter 6, ultraviolet radiation can affect the eyes in many ways. Studies have established that people whose eyes have had a great deal of exposure to UV-B are at greater risk for cataract development, and some studies also indicate that exposure can lead to serious damage to the retina, resulting in age-related macular degeneration. Snow blindness, a reversible condition, is not uncommon among skiers who fail to wear protective eye coverings.

Long before scientific studies confirmed the adverse effects of sunlight on the eyes, different people created ways of shielding the eyes. Natives of the arctic region and Native Americans carved goggles of walrus ivory or wood with narrow slits in them to limit the amount of light that entered their eyes and to protect themselves from snow blindness. Many years ago the Chinese ground lenses from colored pieces of crystal for the same purpose.

Everyone needs sunglasses. The color of your eyes has no bearing on your vulnerability to the sun. The stronger the sun is and the more you are out in it, the greater is your need for protection. Skiers and boaters undergo a great deal of UVR exposure over a long period of time, as do people who spend time on tropical beaches, so they require especially good eye protection. Surfers should wear goggles that screen out ultraviolet radiation. Sunglasses should also be worn when driving in bright sun, because the glare is likely to make you squint, limiting your vision and increasing your risk of having an accident. A typical clear windshield does block a good deal of ultraviolet radiation, however, and a tinted one blocks still more.

People who have had their natural lens removed for treatment of cataracts no longer have the natural protection the lens provides, so they must be especially careful to guard their eyes from ultraviolet radiation. Beginning in the early 1980s, many people who were operated on for cataracts have had an intraocular lens containing compounds that absorb UV light placed in the eye. Anyone who has had cataract surgery or is contemplating it should discuss this option with the ophthalmologist.

Individuals who are undergoing PUVA treatment (which makes use of the photosensitive medication, Psoralen), as described in chapter 2, should wear sunglasses for at least 24 hours after treatment, because of the increased risk of developing cataracts. People being treated with other photosensitizing drugs should take similar precautions.

For your health and comfort and for greater safety when driving or performing any task that requires accurate vision in the sun, you should wear sunglasses. A hat with a brim also provides good protection against ultraviolet radiation.

Questions and Answers About Sunglasses

To help you choose appropriate sunglasses, I have turned to a number of experts: the American Academy of Ophthalmology; the Sunglass Association of America; the American National Standards Institute; the Food and Drug Administration; the Skin Cancer Foundation; Jacqueline Lustgarten, MD, associate clinical professor of ophthalmology at the Mount Sinai School of Medicine; and Dr. Stephen Rozenberg, optometrist at 10/10 Optics. The *Consumer Reports* issue of August 1988 has provided much of the information in written form. The question-and-answer section that follows is a synthesis of these sources.

What do sunglasses do?
They make you much more comfortable in bright sunlight. Sunglasses enhance the eye's normal filtering effects, as well as freeing you from squinting and grimacing. Most important, properly selected sunglasses protect your eyes from the short- and long-range adverse effects of ultraviolet radiation upon your eyes.

What are the different types of light?
Ultraviolet radiation (invisible light) represents only 6 percent of the total quantity of solar energy reaching the earth. The remainder of the energy is composed of infrared rays and visible light rays.

Infrared rays are experienced as heat, and there is no evidence that this energy does the eyes any harm. Visible light, which is perceived by us as colors, is important because it enables us to see objects; however, as we all know, when too much of it strikes our eyes we become uncomfortable. The visible spectrum of light consists of the rainbow of individual hues that combine to form white light. The first wavelength in this visible spectrum is blue-violet light, which many scientists believe can be damaging to the eyes.

What are the effects of blue light?

A number of experts believe that cumulative exposure to blue light may affect the retina and be a factor in developing macular degeneration, a condition in which the functioning of the macula (the high-resolution or fine-tuning part of the retina, needed for close work) grows progressively worse. This condition can eventually result in blindness. Other experts, however, feel that the relationship of blue light to macular degeneration has not yet been satisfactorily established.

Some eyeglass makers promote their products with claims that the lenses block all blue light. But sunglasses that block out all blue light can distort colors, not letting you identify reds as red, greens as green, and blues as blue. Most experts believe that just limiting the blue light is sufficient. General-purpose sunglasses that meet the American National Standards Institute (ANSI) guidelines block at least 75 percent of visible light, thereby providing adequate protection from blue light.

What types of sunglasses offer the best general protection?

Routine protection for the eyes on a sunny day is provided by a lens that lowers the brightness of all wavelengths of light and filters out most invisible ultraviolet radiation and visible blue light.

Until recently, it was difficult for a consumer to evaluate sunglasses in terms of their protection, so many people felt more confident in purchasing an expensive brand or shopping for them at an optical store that also made prescription glasses.

But now, at long last, the Sunglass Association of American (SAA), an industry group, working together with the United States Food and Drug Administration (FDA) has developed and adopted a UV labeling program for rating nonprescription sunglasses and providing consumers with uniform, sound, and useful UV labeling. Because sunglasses are medical devices, they are regulated by the FDA; and both that agency and the SAA were becoming increasingly concerned about the seeming use of scare tactics in the marketplace and, on the other hand, the public's need for eye protection. In 1985 the two groups began preliminary discussions on the issues involved, culminating in a series of meetings in 1988 on the subjects of solar energy and the eye, the role of sunglasses, and sunglass standards.

The voluntary labeling program to be carried out by the SAA is based on the UV categories specified by the American National Standards Institute and was developed by consensus agreement among representatives from the eyecare profession, educators, researchers, the military, other government agencies, and industry; as such, it constitutes the only authoritative document covering the properties and performance of sunglasses. Known as the ANSI Z80.3-1986 Sunglass Standard, it specifies precise standard wording for labels to be placed on a tag or sticker included with each pair of sunglasses.

When the standard was announced in the spring of 1989, FDA Commissioner Frank Young said, "For a long time the FDA has urged people to read food labels and read drug labels. Now we're saying it's important to read information on sunglass labels as well."

The program is planned for implementation by 1992, but as early as the summer of 1989 sunglasses makers were beginning to show that they were taking the guidelines seriously; approved labels were already appearing on many sunglasses found in stores nationwide.

What are the specifics of the SAA labeling program?
The SAA labeling program specifies standard wording on labels in the following form:

"Meets ANSI Z80.3 COSMETIC UV requirements
Blocks at least 70% UVB and 20% UVA."

or

"Meets ANSI Z80.3 GENERAL PURPOSE UV requirements
Blocks at least 95% UVB and 60% UVA."

or

"Meets ANSI Z80.3 SPECIAL PURPOSE UV requirements.
Blocks at least 99% UVB and 60% UVA."

Further, the program also allows the manufacturer or importer-distributor to specify the actual percentage of UV-B and UV-A blocked by the product, beneath the basic policy statement. This additional information, if used, is to be stated in the following form:

"These lenses block XX% UVB and YY% UVA."

To help consumers understand what the labeling means in terms of personal selection and use, the following information on types of sunglasses is also available to consumers:

* *Cosmetic sunglasses* are lightly tinted and are recommended for nonharsh sunlight activities, such as shopping or other around-town uses, out of the direct sun. They block less than 60 percent of visible light, but they block at least 70 percent of UV-B radiation and at least 20 percent of UV-A radiation. These are the least protective sunglasses.
* *General-purpose sunglasses* are recommended for any sunlight activity, such as for beach, boating, driving, flying, hiking, picnicking, and snow use. They are adequate for most uses for most people. General-purpose sunglasses block from 60 percent to 92 percent of visible light, and they block at least 95 percent of UV-B radiation and at least 60 percent of UV-A radiation.
* *Special-purpose sunglasses*, as their label implies, are recommended for special purposes. They may block from as much as 97 percent to as little as 20 percent of visible light. Darker shades are recommended for people who often engage in activities in very bright environments, such as skiing, mountain climbing, or vacationing at a tropical beach. Lighter shades may be preferred in dimmer situations, such as for skiing on overcast days. Special-purpose sunglasses block at least 99 percent of UV-B and 60 percent of UV-A.

Do all sunglasses meet or exceed these guidelines?
Not all sunglasses meet the ANSI guidelines. Remember that these guidelines are voluntary; consequently, you may see nonprescription sunglasses that do not display a label at all. If you do, don't buy them.

On the other hand, some sunglasses may exceed the guidelines. For instance, widely recognized brands such as Bolle, Bausch & Lomb, and Corning, as well as some very moderately priced but less well-known brands, make lenses that claim 100 percent UV-A and UV-B protection. Light transmission varies, depending on the color of the lens, but a given pair of sunglasses should meet or exceed the guidelines for its type, whether costmetic, general-purpose, or special-purpose. Generally, eyecare professionals feel that the ANSI Z80.3-1986 establishes sufficient protection and does not need to be exceeded, although some experts have suggested that the standards should be more stringent.

Are any special style of sunglass frames better than others?

Sunglasses that wrap around or fit closely offer the most protection. Sunglasses with small lenses that sit down about ½ inch from the nose allow roughly 20 percent of the light to reach the eye by seeping in around the lenses, as do larger sunglasses that do not fit close to the face.

In one study it was noted that, if sunglasses do not fit closely, almost three times as much UV radiation reaches the eye as would if they fit correctly. One way to keep light from reaching the eyes around the frames is by using side shields, which are attached to some models.

Sunglasses should be comfortable. When you try them on, make sure that the frame distributes the weight evenly on your nose and that they fit with snug, comfortable pressure behind your ears. Frames can range widely in style and construction, so it is wise to check them carefully before you buy. Hinges should look sturdy, and the ear pieces (temples) should not have too much play, to ensure continued good fit and service.

Do ordinary eyeglasses block ultraviolet radiation?

Most people are surprised to learn that they do. Although they vary in protective capacity, glass lenses generally block a considerable amount of UV light, and plastic lenses block still more. A clear dye coating which absorbs all, or most, UVR can be obtained. Lenses designed for additional UVR absorption or inhibition can also be obtained.

What color should sunglasses be?

The color of the lens and the darkness of the tint are unrelated to their ability to block UVR. Thus, in choosing a color, personal preference may win out; still, experts agree on certain guidelines, as follows.

Trust your eyes to see if the lenses seem too dark or not dark enough. If you are particularly light-sensitive, you may prefer darker lenses or medium ones even in the winter. If you know you will be wearing the glasses at the beach or while skiing, you may want dark lenses; if you just plan to be walking along city streets on sunny summer days, a medium shade is probably just fine. Naturally you won't want your glasses to be so dark that you can't see clearly, but you will want them to be dark enough to save you from squinting, especially if you are driving or engaging in some other activity that requires keen sight.

Some colors can distort reality. Amber glasses, for instance, are excellent for blocking blue light, but they can also make differentiating red from green difficult. If you are considering buying a pair, arrange to go outside the store and look at traffic lights. If you have trouble distinguishing red, green, and yellow, don't buy them. Many people find that brown and brown-amber lenses improve contrast, and they have no problems with them in traffic. Try this out for yourself.

Blue lenses look attractive, but they allow too much blue light to penetrate, so they are not recommended.

Gray lenses are neutral and transmit all colors evenly. Lenses of a brownish or greenish hue are least likely to distort colors, and the light they pass is natural and comfortable. Generally, dark gray or dark green tints permit the most normal color vision. Sunglasses should not make the world look different; rather, they should just block the bright rays of the sun and eliminate glare. And of course, they should block UVR.

Remember, however, that the color of the lenses and the lightness or darkness of that color do not affect their UVR-blocking qualities. For this information, you must depend on the labels.

Is it true that very darkly tinted sunglasses that do not block UVR are worse than no glasses?
Various experts have asserted that dark glasses can make the pupils dilate (open up more), allowing more UVR to reach deeper eye structures. Other experts counter that even very dark sunglasses cause pupils to dilate only slightly. Regardless of this controversy, if you are careful to purchase sunglasses that meet ANSI standards for the purpose for which you plan to wear them, you need not be concerned since little or no UVR will be transmitted. It is also worthy of note that the experts who sounded the alarm did so before the industry began to advise consumers of the amount of UVR protection in each pair of sunglasses.

Are there different types of lenses?
There certainly are, and choosing among them can become confusing. Thus, the following primer on lenses may be helpful:

* *Plain lenses*: Just as the name indicates, these are plain lenses in plastic or high-impact glass, tinted uniformly.
* *Gradient lenses*: These lenses are relatively light at the bottom of the lens and get progressively darker toward the top. Lightly tinted versions are used for fashion glasses, meant to be worn indoors or when there is no sun. Single-gradient sunglasses are

good for driving because they cut overhead glare and still give good vision for the dashboard. Outdoors in bright sun, however, they can be bothersome; as you move your head around, the light seems to change continually.

* *Double-gradient lenses*: These lenses are darker at the top and bottom and lighter in the middle. Many people like them for sports. However, *Consumer Reports* found that they were not good for driving because they dimmed the dashboard more than the view of the road. And as in single-gradient lenses, the differences in shading they create can be annoying when you move your head up and down.

* *Polarizing lenses*: These lenses are especially good for eliminating direct glare and glare reflected from shiny surfaces. Consequently, they are favorites with fishermen, who must constantly look into the water, and with drivers, who must cope with glare that bounces off the road or passing cars.

* *Mirror lenses*: Ideal for unusually intense glare, these lenses feature a thin metallic coating over a regular sunglass lens, creating a mirrored look (usually orange or blue) that adds an extra barrier against glare. Silver-coated mirror lenses are made with very thin metallic coatings and can be applied to plain or gradient-type lenses. They reflect rather than absorb light, thereby effectively reducing glare. Most coatings are vulnerable to scratching, but a scratch-resistant coating can also be applied.

* *Photochromic lenses*: These lenses are very light-sensitive, automatically lightening or darkening in response to the sun's brightness. All-weather photochromic lenses change density and color, depending on both light and temperature, so they are good for all kinds of conditions. They are especially suitable if you are going to be switching from the bright outdoors to shady or indoor areas. However, they can take up to five minutes to lighten (they darken in about half a minute), which can be annoying if you have just come in from outside and are now depending on your prescription lenses in order to see what you are doing! Photochromic lenses are usually acceptable for driving, because they never get extremely dark in the car—since the roof and windows block out much of the outside light. They are especially convenient for people who don't want to carry extra glasses with them.

How can you tell if sunglasses are distortion-free?

Holding the glasses in your hand, look through one lens at a time at a vertical line; then move the glasses back and forth. Next look at a horizontal line, and move the glasses up and down. If the lines either bend or seem distorted, don't buy the glasses.

Vision can also be distorted by frames with wide temples that obstruct peripheral vision. Many sunglasses that have wide sides are just fine for relaxing at the beach but pose a real hazard if you are driving or even walking in busy traffic.

Do lenses come in different materials?

Most sunglasses today are made of plastic, because plastic sunglasses are lighter than glass ones and are more resistant to impact. The FDA requires that all eyeglass lenses, including those for sunglasses, be made of impact-resistant glass or plastic. They are not shatterproof, but they can withstand moderately sharp blows and so are reasonably safe for general use.

Plastic sunglasses require more care than glass ones, because they can easily become scratched. Clean them by rinsing them off with water and then wiping them with a very soft tissue. Be sure not to use a coated tissue; it will add new smudges.

What is the safest, most impact-resistant lens material available?

Polycarbonate is an impact-resistant plastic first introduced in the 1960s for use in bulletproof windows. It is extremely strong and a sensible choice in industrial, hobby, or leisure settings that are likely to involve exposure to flying objects such as materials or a ball. Polycarbonate lenses are tougher and 50 percent lighter than glass lenses; tougher and 10 percent lighter than conventional plastic lenses. Safe as they are, they may not offer you total protection in sports such as racquetball, but they are far less likely to shatter on impact than ordinary plastic glasses. For extra protection, they should be made with material 3 mm thick.

Since polycarbonate lenses block almost all UVR rays, they offer excellent protection, but they are not suitable for every prescription. Even more than regular plastic, they are prone to becoming scratched or pitted, which may distort vision and lessen some of their protective qualities.

Skiers should wear goggles to protect themselves from wind, and it would be wise to get the safe polycarbonate ones, which provide near total protection from UVR.

Are there special coatings for glasses?

Yes. As was stated earlier, clear UV-absorbing coatings are available for everyday prescription glasses. If for some reason you do not want a tint or want to have year-round UVR protection, this is a good idea. If you wear a hat, you may not be bothered by visible light; yet UVR protection is still important. Discuss this with your eyecare professional.

Are tinted glasses good for night driving?
No! Never wear sunglasses at dusk or at night. Many people have the mistaken idea that a yellow tint in their glasses helps brighten up things, but it simply cuts down on the light that enters your eyes. Many cars and trucks have tinted windshields, cutting out some light and providing all the reduction you need. Headlights may bother you, which is why there is a temptation to wear glasses with yellow lenses or a light tint at night. But in cutting back on the light that enters your eyes, you are also reducing the amount of light available to permit you to see vehicles, people, or anything else with which you might collide.

If you are bothered by a reflection off the inside of your regular prescription glasses, you may be tempted to get a tinted pair for night driving. An antireflective coating is a better solution, according to Dr. Stephen Rozenberg, optometrist at New York's 10/10 Optics. This actually increases the amount of light that passes through, thus reducing or eliminating "ghost images."

Do good sunglasses have to be expensive?
Absolutely not. *Consumer Reports* noted only minor differences in UV-reducing qualities between the least expensive and the most expensive ones. The frames, the overall appearance, and distortion-freeness of the lenses may be of superior quality in moderate- or higher-priced glasses, but it is quite possible to find excellent sunglasses for under $15. If you don't need prescription lenses, you may want to have a few pairs of sunglasses on hand—either for different purposes or just to make a fashion statement. Be sure that any sunglasses you buy meet the ANSI requirements for their intended purpose and that a tag or sticker to this effect is included with the glasses.

What's the best approach if you need prescription glasses?
There is really no "best approach," because there are so many individual needs. Your regular prescription glasses block a certain amount of UVR, and they can be treated with chemicals that block still more. This will give you protection but may not meet your needs for comfort, since visible light will still be causing some glare and making

you squint, unless you wear a wide-brimmed hat or visor. For this reason, many people choose to have a pair of sunglasses made up with their prescription.

If you have antireflective coatings (the same kind used on good camera lenses and binoculars to improve clarity and reduce glare) added to your regular prescription lenses, you will find that glare is minimized but that the glasses still do not substitute for sunglasses. These coated lenses are most useful if you have poor night vision or if you work in an environment with low light. Such coatings, despite their glare-reducing qualities, can increase the amount of light transmitted through lenses from 92 percent to almost 100 percent, yet they do not transmit any additional ultraviolet radiation.

If you generally stay out of the sun or only wear eyeglasses for reading, you may prefer to have one pair of nonprescription sunglasses and one pair of clip-on lenses that you slip over your prescription glasses. Far less expensive than buying a second pair of glasses, these clip-ons should meet the appropriate ANSI standards and should be so labeled.

If you wear eyeglasses for driving, you may prefer the clip-ons for occasions when the sun suddenly dims or when you go through a tunnel; in these instances, rather than having to change glasses, you can simply flip up the clip-ons. Before buying them, discuss this option with your optician, because some plastic lenses (especially those with antireflective coatings) are easily scratched and so may not be compatible with clip-ons.

Do contact lenses block UVR?

Some do, but not all of them block a sufficient quantity of it. Discuss this with your eyecare professional. Generally speaking, you are better off to wear sunglasses over your contacts: it will give you more protection and will save you from having to squint when the visible light hits your eyes.

Should children wear sunglasses?

It's a good idea, but the sunglasses must be made of a totally safe material if children are going to be running and playing in them. Many experts believe that children's glasses should, whenever possible, be made of polycarbonate.

The natural lens in a young child's eye is somewhat transparent to UVR, so the eye needs extra protection. But unless sunlight is very strong—for example, if the child is fishing, skiing, or traveling in the tropics—a baseball hat with a brim may provide sufficient sun protection.

Because the potential for cumulative damage to a child's eyes is so great from exposure to UVR, numerous experts have stated that eye protection is an essential part of preventive care, on a par with immunization and early dental care.

Do I need to wear sunglasses every time I venture out into the sun?

No, not unless you feel especially sensitive to the sun. When braving the midday summer sun, when driving on a glary day, while skiing, and certainly when exposed to the sun for extended periods of time, you need this protection. Use good sense: if you are squinting, you need them; if you are wearing a hat that protects your eyes and you are not engaging in an activity that involves much sun exposure, you may be able to leave them in your pocket or bag. But don't leave your sunglasses home, since weather (like your schedule of activities) has a way of changing after you go out.

Can I depend on sunglasses to protect me at all times?

Even sunglasses that claim to eliminate 100 percent of ultraviolet radiation will not protect you if you continue to stare directly at the sun or at an eclipse. Similarly, they will not protect you against artificial light sources such as ultraviolet lamps or lamps in tanning booths. (See chapter 3 for facts about tanning salons and artificial tanning.) For these purposes, you need totally opaque goggles.

What are the best sunglasses to get?

The best sunglasses are those that protect you from ultraviolet radiation and visible light. Beyond that, you need to decide which kind best suits your lifestyle; and only you know the specific uses to which you will put them.

Do they need to be attractive? Not unless that's important to you.

Should they be comfortable? Of course.

Ruth Domber, owner of 10/10 Optics says it best: "If you are comfortable in glasses, and you like how you look in them, you'll wear them. Glasses that are in your dresser drawer or lying in a case on your desk won't do you any good, no matter what stringent guidelines they meet."

Other Kinds of Protection

Another good source of eye protection against the sun, according to Hugh R. Taylor, MD, associate professor of ophthalmology at the Wilmer Eye Institute of the Johns Hopkins School of Medicine, and his colleagues is a simple brimmed cap. These researchers found that such a cap can cut ocular exposure to UV-B by half, and that the wearing of ordinary glasses with plastic lenses may reduce it to about 5 percent. To minimize ocular exposure to UV-B, people should wear a brimmed hat and close-fitting sunglasses with UV-B-absorbing lenses.

Summary

Studies show that both visible and ultraviolet light can be harmful to the eyes. Bright sunlight can cause temporary and long-lasting damage, and UV-B has been statistically linked to the development of cataracts. Sunglasses are your best defense against all of these effects. Moreover, it is essential that eyes be protected during protracted periods in the sun and under special conditions such as skiing, lounging on a sunny beach, or wading or swimming in the water. Sunglasses that filter out both visible blue light and invisible UVR offer the most protection. A voluntary labeling program has recently been developed by the FDA and the Sunglass Association of America, using guidelines promulgated by the American National Standards Institute (ANSI); these guidelines can help you choose the appropriate sunglasses for your particular needs.

Even the best-quality sunglasses will only offer protection if they fit correctly—and you wear them! Various types and colors of lenses are available, although there is general agreement that dark gray or dark green tints permit the most normal color vision with the least distortion. Price is not an indicator of the ability of a pair of sunglasses to absorb ultraviolet radiation. Thus, excellent protective glasses may be found at the lower end of the price range, and some expensive fashion glasses may offer little protection. The FDA requires that all lenses (prescription and sunglass) be made of impact-resistant glass or plastic. For sports enthusiasts and active children, however, lenses made of polycarbonate are a wise choice. Use common sense and the new ANSI guidelines when you shop for sunglasses.

It is unwise to wear tinted lenses for night driving. Although they may help eliminate the glare of oncoming headlights, they also reduce your night vision to an unacceptable level and thus pose an unnecessary driving risk.

A hat with a brim offers significant protection from UVR all by itself. It also enhances eye protection in conjunction with sunglasses or prescription glasses treated with clear UV-absorbing coatings.

Protecting your eyes against the effects of the sun not only offers a major health advantage, but it can help you avoid the small "age lines" that develop as a result of prolonged squinting.

III

Repairing the Effects of the Sun

12 *Treating Sun-related Eye Conditions*

Many conditions can adversely affect the eyes as a direct or indirect result of sun exposure. Prevention, of course, constitutes the best countermeasure, but self-reproach after the fact is self-defeating. Treatment is available.

Acute conditions such as snow blindness are definitely related to UVR exposure. According to some estimates, about 10 percent of cataracts may be directly related to exposure to ultraviolet radiation; most others are age-related, although it is possible to develop cataracts at any age. Macular degeneration is likely to occur sometime after the age of fifty and generally is not preventable, but it has been linked to UVR exposure. Damage to the conjunctiva may also occur as the result of UVR exposure; and both melanoma on the eyelid and intraocular melanoma are directly associated with exposure to the sun.

Following is a brief review of each condition, together with a description of the treatment that you can expect to receive for it.

Snow Blindness

Snow blindness, or sunburn of the eyes, is the direct and immediate result of UVR exposure, although (as with typical sunburn) symptoms may not show up until 4 to 24 hours after exposure. Its name derives from the concentrated reflection of sunlight off white snow, which can cause it. However, surfers, water-skiers, and anyone else who risks unprotected intense exposure to UVR (including workers who use welding or carbon arc torches) are vulnerable to it, as well. Symptoms may range from mild irritation to severe pain and spasms of the eyelid.

Generally the effects of snow blindness (scientific term: *keratoconjunctivitis*) are temporary and self-limiting, which means that the condition will probably clear up without treatment; but occasionally the cornea remains scarred, especially if the condition is the result of exposure to an artificial source of UVR such as a tanning booth.

Snow blindness can be agonizingly painful, since the cornea feels as if it had been severely scratched. The reason for the pain is that the epithelium (covering) of the cornea has come off. It will grow back, in 24 to 48 hours, however, and in 4 or 5 days it will be as healthy as if nothing had ever happened. Still, anyone suffering from an acute case of snow blindness would be wise to consult an opthalmologist; this specialist may have to administer a local anesthesia (eyedrops) before conducting an examination.

Treatment sometimes consists of eyepatching with antibiotic drops or ointment, which allows the eyes to rest and recover. Alternatively, the doctor may prescribe oral pain relievers or medication to dilate the pupils and relax the eye muscles, in addition to antibiotics.

Cataracts

A cataract is a cloudiness of the lens of the eye. As you will recall from chapter 6, the front window of the eye is the clear cornea. Behind it is the iris, the colored portion of the eye. The pupil is the small round black opening through which light enters; and behind the pupil is a small transparent lens, which changes the focus of the eye, enabling you to see things at different distances.

The lens is normally clear, but with aging (and in some instances, earlier in life) it begins to yellow, and vision becomes less clear. The yellowing can become severe, clouding the lens so that light rays cannot easily pass through, thus diminishing vision. If left untreated, the lens may become completely brown and then opaque.

Cataracts can be diagnosed by an eyecare specialist during an examination with an instrument that lights the inside of the eye. If a cataract develops in one eye, another usually develops in the other eye, too. Some cataracts are so slow-developing that decades may pass before they become severe enough to require action. The only way to remove the cloudy lens is by surgery. Eye drops, salves, and medicines cannot treat cataracts, although considerable research is being done in this area. Sometimes eyeglasses help increase vision; medication that dilates the pupil can also alleviate the problem for a short period of time.

Need for Cataract Surgery

At one time, cataract surgery was delayed until the entire lens had hardened—sometimes referred to as "maturing" or "ripening." It is no longer necessary to wait, however: cataracts can be removed whenever vision is so impaired that it interferes with a person's ability to function in normal daily life. Of course, people's idea of "normal functioning" may differ; and a jeweler, surgeon, draftsman, tailor, hobbyist, or other person who does fine work may require keener vision than others. When a cataract interferes with your ability to drive, work, or function during leisure, surgery is possible. You can decide if you want to have it done then or if you want to wait until symptoms worsen or until the procedure fits your schedule.

Methods of Cataract Surgery

Cataract surgery has not only become more streamlined and efficient in the last few years, but it has also become so safe that it is regularly performed on people over the age of ninety.

The three basic methods of surgery for cataracts are intracapsular, extracapsular, and phacoemulsification. All require an incision into the eye, and all involve a recovery period. However, long hospital stays are no longer indicated for any of these methods, and most people do not even stay overnight in the hospital. We will consider each main type of cataract surgery in turn.

Intracapsular Extraction

The standard method of cataract surgery, in use for about fifty years, involves removal of the entire lens with capsule intact, all in one piece. This used to be accomplished by means of tiny forceps. Today, a freezing probe is usually used to extract the cataract. After an incision is made into the eye near the margin of the iris, a pencillike instrument called a *cryoprobe* is inserted. The cataract adheres to the probe via an iceball, facilitating its removal. With this method both the capsule and the lens are removed, leaving nothing behind that might later become cloudy and cause "after cataracts."

Extracapsular Extraction

In this method, the opaque portion of the lens (the cataract) is removed in parts, without disturbing the posterior capsule, which is left behind. This leaves the other structures in the eye in a more normal position, providing support for the implantation of intraocular lenses (described in the next section) and perhaps offering the retina protection against possible complications. The clear capsule that remains behind the lens sometimes becomes cloudy later on. If this should occur anytime from a few weeks to several years later, the capsule can be removed by means of a burst of energy from a YAG (yttrium-aluminum-garnet) laser. This is performed as an office procedure. Far less frequently under these circumstances, a second small operation is performed to open up the back of the capsule.

Phacoemulsification and Aspiration

This technique for removing a cataract is sometimes referred to as a "laser method," but it doesn't use true laser light; instead, it utilizes ultrasound technology. It requires only a very small incision in the eye. The cataract is broken up into very small pieces while still inside the eye, and then is sucked out with a vibrating titanium needle through the tiny incision. Many opthalmologists have been trained in this newer method, so it is an available option. However, not all patients are candidates for such surgery. If the internal support of the lens has become weakened because of age or injury, phacoemulsification is not likely to be recommended.

Cataract surgery may be performed under either local anesthesia (by injection) or general anesthesia. Either way, it is a painless procedure that involves little or no postoperative discomfort. At one time, patients had to remain still—even in bed—for a substantial period of time afterward, but now the sutures (stitches) used are so improved that people can be up and on their way in no time.

Vision After Cataract Surgery

Those ugly "Coke-bottle-thick" glasses once worn by cataract patients are seldom used today. Aside from their cosmetic drawbacks, they had other disadvantages. The thick lenses magnified images so much that, if only one eye had been operated upon, it was impossible for the brain to integrate the images from both eyes. The glasses were fine for long-distance or close work; but when the wearer tried to focus on something at mid-distance, things seemed to jump in front of them, in what Dr. Jacqueline Lustgarten calls the "jack-in-the-box phenomenon." In addition, these glasses did not allow for good peripheral vision.

Contact lenses overcame some of these problems. Because such lenses magnify images far less, the discrepancy between the images received by both eyes can usually be managed by the brain. In addition, peripheral vision is preserved. Some contact lenses can be worn for extended periods, representing a big improvement over glasses for many patients.

Today, most people have an intraocular lens (IOL) implanted in the eye immediately after the cataract is removed. The IOL is a small, plastic lens placed within the eye to restore the focusing power that had been provided by the eye before the cataract developed. Even with an implant, it is often necessary to correct vision further with ordinary eyeglasses—if not for general use, then for close work.

Initially, the implants were only recommended for the elderly, because the IOL had not yet been proved to last for many years. Now, however, they are so vastly improved and have such a good record for longevity, safety, and effectiveness that people of all ages have this procedure done. Still, many opthalmologists feel that it should not be used on patients under the age of fifty.

In most instances, IOLs are UVR-absorbent, providing some protection against the sun. Be sure to discuss this with your opthalmologist prior to surgery (or if you have already had surgery, find out whether a UVR-absorbent lens was implanted). It is still wise to wear sunglasses in the sun even if your IOL is UVR-absorbent, but it is crucial to do so if your IOL is not.

Complications associated with cataract extraction and intraocular lens implantation are relatively infrequent, but occasionally infections, bleeding, retinal detachment, dislocation of the implant, or glaucoma do arise. In such cases, the problem can usually be managed successfully by the opthalmologist.

Macular Degeneration

Although the condition called *macular degeneration* is most often age-related and has a tendency to run in families, some studies have indicated that UVR exposure may also be implicated. The retina is the thin, light-sensitive tissue that lines the interior of the eye. The macula is the high-resolution or fine-tuning part of the retina, needed for close work. The middle of the macula is responsible for central vision, and when it is damaged or diseased, central vision begins to blur.

Macular degeneration is the most common cause of legal blindness in the United States. The condition tends to sneak up on older people, but early treatment can be extremely helpful. Macular degeneration can be detected by an opthalmologist even before symptoms begin—another good reason for regular checkups.

In most people who suffer from this condition, the macula gets thinner and its cells degenerate. In about 10 percent of all cases, leakage occurs from small blood vessels that grow in the macular region between the retina and its supporting layer of tissue, and this damages the retinal cells responsible for central vision. New and abnormal blood vessels may form in the same area, leading to a further decline in vision.

Formerly, little could be done for this progressively worsening condition; but since the early 1980s, opthalmologists have developed a good treatment for patients whose damage began with the abnormal leakage of blood from the macular vessels. Using a krypton laser light, they pinpoint and beam high-energy light to seal off these blood vessels, deterring new ones from forming. Used when symptoms first appear, this procedure can reduce or slow vision loss in some people. Unfortunately, the treatment is only successful in a small percentage of cases.

The peripheral or side vision of people with macular degeneration is not affected, so they can get around independently. With the aid of large-type reading materials, bright lights, magnifying lenses, and other adaptations, individuals afflicted with the condition can still enjoy a high quality of life. Vitamins, drugs, and particular diets have not yet shown any evidence of halting or reversing macular degeneration, but experiments and research are being conducted on the possible benefits of vitamin E.

Successful preventive methods have not been established, but UVR has been shown to contribute to macular deterioration, so this is another reason to avoid excessive exposure of the eyes to UVR.

Damage to the Conjunctiva

Pinguecula and Pterygia

The conjunctiva—the protective membrane that lines the eyelids and covers the eyeball—can develop benign growths or thickening as a result of cumulative and excessive exposure to ultraviolet radiation. This in turn can lead to pinguecula, a condition in which a triangular, yellowish-white patch appears on either side of the cornea. Finally, pinguecula can lead to pterygia, in which a thick, winglike bit of tissue extends from the nasal border of the cornea toward the middle of the eye.

Pinguecula is cosmetically unattractive, and if growth is directed inward (close to the center of the cornea) it can threaten to impair vision. Generally no treatment is advised, but if the condition is disfiguring or vision is impaired, surgery can be performed to shave the pterygia off the cornea. Pterygia sometimes recurs after initial removal, in which case surgery may be repeated or radiation or medication may be attempted.

Cancer of the Conjunctiva

Although quite rare, cancer of the conjunctiva does occur, usually among older people. Generally slow growing, these cancers may arise from precancerous pigmented tumors. They can deeply invade the layers of the lids, and treatment depends on the type of cancer and the extent of invasion. Such cancers are closely related to the basal cell carcinomas that often develop on skin. Malignant melanoma of the conjunctiva is extremely rare, but it can occur. In this instance, removal of the eye may be necessary.

Treatment may consist of surgical removal of the cancer, radiation therapy, or chemosurgery (better known as Mohs surgery, and described more fully in chapter 14), in combination with follow-up care. Basal cell cancers of the conjunctiva usually respond well to treatment, especially if diagnosed and treated early. Some rarer forms of cancer of the conjunctiva are more difficult to treat, but in most instances vision is preserved even when the surgery involved is extensive.

Cancer of the Eyelid

As a result of UVR exposure, the incidence of cancer of the eyelid has doubled in only ten years. Many cancers that appear on the upper lid are the same kind that develop on the skin: basal cell carcinomas, or the more aggresive (and harder to cure) squamous cell carcinomas. Cancers may also arise in the meibomian glands—structures on the eyelid that produce sebum, an oily secretion. Those that grow on the upper lid progress slowly but can spread beyond the original site; those that arise on the lower lid are less likely to spread.

Removal of small lesions is often just an office procedure; the cancer is simply "shaved" off. There is seldom any loss of vision, and recovery is usually uneventful. But if the cancer has gone undiagnosed or untreated and has grown, surgery may be quite extensive. Eyelashes sometimes fall out or are removed, and tear ducts may be affected, resulting in either constant tearing or dry eyes. After such surgery, artificial eyelashes may be worn for comfort and protection. Sometimes an entire eyelid reconstruction may be necessary. This should be performed by an opthalmic plastic surgeon for best results, using skin grafts from the other lid or from the mouth if necessary. It may be done in two stages, several weeks apart.

If the cancer has gone untreated for a long time and has grown to a large size, the entire eye and the soft tissue around it may have to be removed.

Once again, protection from UVR can help prevent these cancers. Early diagnosis and treatment are essential.

Intraocular Melanoma

Intraocular malignant melanoma is the most common malignant tumor to arise in the eyes of adults in the United States and Europe. Studies demonstrate a strong relationship between melanoma incidence and exposure. Malignant intraocular melanoma is rarely associated with melanoma of the skin, and skin melanomas do not usually spread to the eye.

As discussed in chapter 8, malignant melanoma of the eye usually begins in the melanocytes of the iris, in the ciliary body, or in the choroid.

When malignant melanoma develops in the iris, unlike in other parts of the body, it tends to be slow-growing, and the opthalmologist may appropriately wish to observe it for a short time. If it grows, removal of the tumor (often done during a biopsy) may be all that is needed to effect a cure.

Melanomas that develop on the choroid are far more serious and can metastasize (spread) to other parts of the body. Sometimes the cancer develops near the macula, in which case the first symptom may be a decrease in vision that sends the sufferer off to an eyecare professional. Frequently, however, there are no early symptoms; although it may be noted during a regular eye examination. Sometimes a melanoma on the choroid is not diagnosed until after the cancer has spread to another part of the body.

Treatments for melanomas on the choroid or ciliary body are individualized for each patient, depending on many factors. There is also some controversy as to which treatment is generally optimum. Surgical removal of the eye (enucleation) may be recommended, especially if the tumor has already destroyed vision. However, concern has been expressed by some experts that removal of the eye can lead to spread of the tumor through the vascular system. Alternatively, radiation may be recommended, either by directing radiation to the eye from an external source or by temporarily sewing plaques of radiation to the outside of the eye over the tumor, permitting the radioactive materials to release radiation into the tumor at a predetermined rate. Shrinkage or disappearance of the tumor can be achieved with radiation because it damages both the tumor cells and the blood vessels that supply the tumor. Vision is most often preserved with this treatment.

If intraocular melanoma spreads to other parts of the body, chemotherapy may be indicated. Chemotherapy consists of the use of one or more drugs in combination that can reach all parts of the body, interfering with and destroying cancer cell growth.

Other Cancers of the Eye

Other cancers in other parts of the eye, such as the orbit or eye socket, may affect children or adults; but because they have not been linked to exposure to ultraviolet radiation, we will not discuss them here. These cancers, like the ones described previously, respond well to treatment, and cure rates are good.

Altogether, about 2,500 new cases of eye cancer are reported each year, and about 400 deaths from this cause occur annually. As in all instances of a serious medical problem, it is often wise to get a second opinion before embarking on a prescribed program of treatment. An opthalmologist who has special training and experience in treating cancer should always be consulted.

Summary

Exposure to ultraviolet radiation has been linked to certain age-related conditions of the eye, particularly cataracts and macular degeneration. Cataract surgery today has been greatly improved and simplified, and results are usually excellent. A small proportion of people with macular degeneration have responded well to laser treatment, but generally little can be done for it. However, peripheral vision is usually spared, so individuals with this condition can still lead a reasonably normal life.

The cornea can be temporarily but painfully affected by severe exposure to UVR, resulting in snow blindness. Although this clears up quickly, it often requires medical attention. The conjunctiva responds to excessive UVR by developing benign growths that may be cosmetically unattractive and in some instances may impair vision. These growths can safely be removed. Cancer of the conjunctiva, the eyelid, and the eye itself are also linked to UVR exposure. These cancers, including melanoma, respond well to various treatments—radiation, chemotherapy, and surgery—if treated in a timely fashion. In most instances, vision is preserved.

13 *Treating Sun-Damaged Skin*

Most of us grew up under the influence of a number of health warnings: don't go out in the rain without your raingear; if someone on the bus or in the movies is coughing, move away; stay out of the ocean when the waves are too rough. The list is endless, with some strictures having more validity than others. Unfortunately, we were also told to "get some sun", in order to avoid contracting rickets or simply to be suffused in those seemingly beneficial rays. Few people ever heard that the sun could damage their skin, prematurely aging it or causing cancer.

During our growing-up years, most of us didn't listen to any advice. Later, when I would regret this inattention, my mother, in her infinite wisdom, would say, "Don't cry over spilt milk. Just mop it up."

There is nothing to be gained from rehashing old behaviors. By now you know all about the effects of the sun on your body, and you know how to be safe in the sun; still, you will want to know what can be done to treat and (in some instances) to reverse the damage already done.

It is easy to confuse natural aging with *photoaging*, the term for skin changes that occur only in skin exposed to significant amounts of sun or other sources of ultraviolet radiation. There are a number of differences, however, and the two kinds of skin changes are biologically separate events. Natural aging is a condition in which there is a deepening of normal expression lines and a loss of elasticity and thickness of skin. In photoaging the skin may have deep wrinkles; be coarse, parched looking, thickened, and leathery; and lack elasticity. Telangiectasia (fishnetlike display of "broken" blood vessels), mottled irregular pigmentation, brown age spots, solar lentigines (brown flat spots on the backs of hands and on the face), actinic or solar keratoses (smooth, flat or slightly raised pink spots that become irregular, scaly, and wartlike and turn darker—and have a strong potential for moving on to become squamous cell carcinomas) may all be present.

All of the above are treatable and in some instances reversible.

Heatstroke and Sunburn

In heatstroke and sunstroke, body temperature can rise to a dangerously high level. This is an emergency that can be fatal. First aid for heatstroke consists of quick cooling. Application of an ice bag or crushed ice, or even wrapping in a wet sheet or hosing down with cold water will help while someone calls the local medics or arranges to get the victim to an emergency room.

Sunburns may happen—if not to you (since you are careful!), then to someone you know. Mild sunburns can usually be treated with an assortment of nonprescription sunburn preparations. These often contain a local anesthetic and are available in various forms: liquid, cream, ointment, aerosol, and pump spray. The alcohol included in some of these products cools the skin but may cause further irritation on sunburned skin. Read directions carefully. Generally these non-prescription medications work well on small areas, but if applied to most of the exposed area (such as 50 percent of the body surface) or if applied more than four times daily, they can be absorbed into the body, causing toxicity. Most sunburn remedies should be kept away from the eyes and should not be used if the skin is broken, raw, or blistered. In the event of a severe sunburn or symptoms that worsen or persist more than a few days, or if any sign of infection or increased swelling appears, medical attention should be sought.

When a sunburn begins to heal, the skin tends to feel dry and rough. A good moisturizing lotion or petroleum jelly applied to it will help keep the skin moist and will minimize or even avoid peeling. Other treatments for sunburn include soaking in either a cool plain bath or one to which Burrow's solution or oatmeal has been added. Sunburn raises the temperature of the skin, increasing the damage already done by the sun. Cooling the skin minimizes the damage. In addition cool water works like an anesthetic, quelling the pain, and it subdues swelling and inflammation. Pat rather than rub the skin dry, using a clean towel.

Aspirin, ibuprofen, and acetaminophen are all useful in alleviating pain from sunburn. Many doctors suggest taking two aspirin or ibuprofen after sun exposure, repeating the dose every two hours for the next twelve hours to avoid the discomfort of a severe sunburn.

Photoaging Treatments

Many of the results of photoaging do not pose health threats, but they can have an adverse emotional effect on people. In a society that values good looks and youth, no one wants to have unnecessary acquired cosmetic flaws or to look old prematurely. There is no reason to endure unsightly photoaging, if it is making you unhappy. Fortunately, much can be done about this. When sun exposure is completely avoided for a number of years, a layer of new collagen (a protein that, along with elastin, is responsible for the support and elasticity of the skin) appears in the dermis, causing the skin to begin to appear younger and more attractive. A number of safe and efficacious methods can contribute significantly to making your skin look the way it should.

Techniques and medical methods to treat photoaging vary; options include dermabrasion, cryosurgery, electrosurgery, chemical peels, 5-fluorouracil (5-FU) treatments, collagen injections, plastic surgery, and (newest of all) the use of tretinoin, also known as Retin-A®. All of these procedures should be performed or supervised by an experienced physician, preferably a board-certified dermatologist or plastic surgeon.

Dermabrasion

Dermabrasion is a technique of skin abrasion or burning that is performed with a motor-driven, high-speed tool. It has come a long way since it was first introduced in the 1950s. Today, the abrading device looks a bit like a miniature sanding tool, and indeed it does sand or plane the skin.

Prior to the procedure, patients are usually given an intravenous painkiller and a mild sedative to help them relax and avoid pain. Then, section by section, the skin is frozen by application of an aerosol freeze spray. This simultaneously firms up the skin, facilitating the planing, and numbs the skin. Then the physician takes the rapidly rotating brush and strokes it across the face to remove the upper layers of the skin. Some patients say that the procedure is painful, and for this reason general anesthesia may be used. Others say that only the spray of blood and skin bothered them. The face is bandaged afterward, but the patient usually removes the bandages at home.

To reduce swelling, patients are advised to keep their heads elevated the first few nights. Painkillers and antibiotics are prescribed for the period of convalescence. Crusting, intense redness, and swelling develop in the abraded skin within 24 to 48 hours. Within two weeks, the crusts shed, leaving the skin thinner but still pinkish red, with the color gradually diminishing within a few months. People usually need to take two weeks off from work or social activities following dermabrasion. Sun exposure must be avoided during this time, so a sunscreen or other protection should be worn even for brief outings in the sun.

Dermabrasion is most often used to treat acne scars, but it has also been successfully used to treat other scars and actinic keratoses of the face and scalp. It is more successful on fair-skinned individuals than on those with dark or olive complexions, because the latter are at greater risk of developing hyperpigmentation (areas of darkened skin). Advocates of this treatment say that skin texture is improved, wrinkling is reduced, and mottled skin is replaced by more supple skin of nearly uniform color. They also say that it helps prevent recurrence of actinic keratoses for at least four years; and with careful protection from the sun, this time can be extended. Authorities who are less enthusiastic about this technique for actinic keratoses state that the lesions may recur within eight months of dermabrasion.

Dermabrasion carries some risk for infections, scarring, and permanent skin discoloration. Because it is a slow, painstaking procedure that requires much skill, it should only be performed by a physician specially trained and experienced in the technique.

Chemical Peels

Sometimes referred to as *chemabrasion,* a chemical peel involves application of a caustic chemical material to the face. This material destroys the top layer (or layers) of the skin, causing it (or them) to slough off and permitting the growth of new, fresh skin. Chemical peels, unlike other treatments for photoaged skin, are only done on the face, because the procedure might scar other areas such as the arms or hands.

There are two kinds of chemical peels: trichloracetic acid (TCA), often referred to as a *superficial* or *light peel;* and phenol. TCA is used to treat light wrinkling, sun damage, and irregular pigmentation. The greater the amount of sun damage, the stronger the solution used. The procedure takes about an hour to perform if the entire face is done, and it causes little or no pain. An anti-anxiety medication may be given prior to the procedure, but usually only a mild pain medication is needed. The physician applies the TCA solution with cotton-tipped applicators. When application is completed, a white frost develops on the face, and is then rinsed off with cold water or alcohol. Some physicians tape the face, in a process called *occlusion,* which keeps air from reaching the treated area, thus prolonging the activity of the ingredients and increasing the depth of the peel.

A TCA chemical peel doesn't remove deep wrinkles or those near the mouth, but it may reduce moderate wrinkles, and it often fades solar lentigines and freckles. The effect on pigmentation is unpredictable, however, and nevi often get darker.

Phenol peels are stronger than TCA peels and are more likely to be used for actinic keratoses. They may be used over the entire face or just in small areas such as around the mouth. Because phenol peels can cause some systemic side effects, they are not appropriate for individuals with chronic kidney disease or liver disease. Cardiac arrhythmias occasionally occur during a full phenol peel, so for this reason physicians should monitor the patient's heart with a continuous EKG during the procedure.

Sedation and painkillers are administered prior to a phenol peel, and the procedure follows much the same steps as are used for the lighter TCA peel. The chemical formula most often used includes phenol, cotton oil, liquid soap, and distilled water.

Following either kind of peel, there is some swelling and a feeling of tightness, warmth, and pain. Later, the skin itches. A hard crust and scabs eventually form, although some physicians may recommend the use of antibiotic creams immediately after the peel, in order to reduce or avoid the hard crusts. The scabs loosen after seven to ten days and fall off, leaving a layer of very pink skin that heals and forms new skin.

Following a chemical peel, it is essential to avoid the sun. On occasions when it is impossible to stay out of the sun during the next few months, a total sunblock must be used.

Sometimes hyperpigmentation occurs in the treated area, particularly in dark-skinned people, so many physicians feel this technique is best suited to patients with light skin. It is always possible that skin color may differ between treated and surrounding skin. Occasionally, scarring occurs, particularly if the solution penetrates too deeply.

Chemical peels should never be administered by nonmedical personnel; only an experienced physician should perform it.

Cryosurgery

Cryosurgery—whose prefix *cryo*, means "icy cold" or "frost" in Greek—is a form of surgery that makes use of subzero temperatures to destroy tissue. In one form of cryosurgery, solid carbon dioxide or liquid nitrogen is applied to a growth with a sterile cotton-tipped applicator or is sprayed directly onto the skin. A blister then forms, which is followed by necrosis (death) of the tissue. The procedure can be repeated if necessary, either at this time or at a later session.

In other forms of cryosurgery, a freezing chemical is circulated through a metal probe, which is then applied to the unwanted growth. The tissues freeze when they adhere to the cold metal of the probe, and the cell membranes burst, killing the cells, which are then sloughed off. Underlying structures are not affected. Stitches or bandaging is not needed, and healing is usually uneventful. Scarring seldom occurs, but sometimes hyperpigmentation surrounds the lesion, and depigmentation can occur at the lesion site. The hyperpigmentation is usually temporary, but the depigmentation can be permanent.

Cryosurgery can be used to treat various sun-induced conditions such as solar lentigines, actinic keratoses, and skin cancers. It can be used on any part of the face (including the eyelids), on the hands, and on any other part of the body. Often, lentigines and actinic keratoses are treated by contact with cryoprobes cooled by nitrous oxide gas or with cotton-tipped wooden applicators dipped in liquid nitrogen. Many physicians prefer to spray the liquid nitrogen evenly over the surface of the lesion until it turns completely white, with the whiteness extending beyond the margins of the lesion.

There is no pain during the procedure, but discomfort or pain may develop later. After the problem areas are frozen, hivelike skin eruptions may occur nearby, and later a brown crust forms that may exude some fluid. The lesions separate and fall off in seven to ten days.

Complications or postoperative infections are rare, and cryosurgery is safe even for people with other medical problems.

Surgery: Excisional, Curettage, Electrosurgery, and Plastic

Some small precancerous growths, such as actinic keratoses, benign nevi, and dysplastic nevi may be removed surgically, usually in the dermatologist's office. This may be done for the purpose of biopsy (as described in chapter 7) as a form of treatment, or for cosmetic reasons. The physician uses a scalpel blade or a curette (a spoon- or scoop-shaped instrument) to remove the growth. The edges of the skin may or may not be sutured (stitched). Local anesthesia is usually all that is necessary for the procedure; occasionally a pain reliever may be prescribed for postoperative discomfort or pain.

Electrosurgery makes use of surgical instruments that operate on a high-frequency current. In electrocoagulation, the physician uses a needle or snare to destroy tissue. This technique is sometimes referred to as *electric cautery* or *galvanocautery*. It is used to remove moles, growths, brown spots, and discolorations, as well as actinic keratoses and skin cancers.

Electrodesiccation, also called *fulguration,* is another form of electrosugery. Here, tissue is destroyed by being burned with an electric spark. This technique is suitable for eliminating small superficial growths and for aiding in curettage. The procedure helps to destroy and dry up unwanted growths. The wounds heal well by themselves without any stitches. It may be used for various sun-related growths, particularly telangiectasia on the face. Occasionally, tiny scars may remain where the needle was placed; but if a minimum amount of current is used, such scarring is less likely to occur. This is another reason for choosing an experienced physician.

Although there are various ways to minimize wrinkles, a surgical face-lift is the only way to eliminate sagging skin. This surgery consists of trimming away excess skin and pulling the rest of the facial skin slightly tighter. Deep furrows on the brow can be eliminated similarly, by trimming away and tightening the skin. The procedure is performed by a plastic surgeon.

A blepharoplasty, which works in much the same way as a face-lift, eliminates sagging eyelids that may be impeding vision and causing distress about appearance. It is performed by a plastic surgeon or by an opthalmologist who has special training in plastic surgery.

Many people choose to have various defects—congenital or acquired, sun-related or not—surgically corrected. Either dermatologists or plastic surgeons can remove unsightly growths, but changes in contours of chins, jaws, and noses, as well as face-lifts and blepharoplasties, fall within the realm of plastic surgery.

Collagen Replacement

Collagen is a protein in the body that helps to support the skin and other soft tissues. As was explained in chapter 2, elastin and collagen fibers are part of the connective and elastic tissue in the dermis, the layer beneath the epidermis. Age and sun damage break down this tissue, causing sagging and wrinkles. Most people have heard about collagen, perhaps because so many expensive cosmetics include it in their ingredients. But collegen cannot be absorbed through the skin in cream or ointment form. On the other hand, it *can* be implanted.

The collagen used in implantation is a natural animal protein made from the skin of cattle. It is injected through a small hypodermic needle, filling in skin depressions such as those caused by wrinkles.

Approved by the FDA in 1981, Zyderm® collagen implants have been demonstrated to be safe and effective. They are available in three forms: Zyderm® I, the original product; Zyderm® II, introduced in 1983; and Zyplast, introduced in 1985. Acne, surgical and trauma scars, and wrinkles (whether age-related or sun-induced) generally are greatly improved by these purified bovine collagen injections, performed by a dermatologist or plastic surgeon.

Generally, a person's state of health is not a limiting factor in considering this procedure. However, anyone with a history of auto-immune disease, such as lupus or rheumatoid arthritis, or severe allergic reactions should not undergo the procedure. The physician will test for allergies to the material by injecting a small amount of collagen into the forearm 28 days before the planned procedure. The test site is then observed 72 hours later and again 4 weeks later. For added safety, the doctor may test the patient again, this time using the forearm or forehead as the test site. The double testing technique reduces the chance of causing a serious adverse treatment reaction.

If all goes well in the testing, an appointment is made for the collagen injections. It takes only a few moments to perform the procedure; injections are done at one time, but depending on the extent of the wrinkling, several sessions may be necessary. There is little or no discomfort associated with the injections, and people can return to their usual activities immediately afterward.

The benefits of collagen injections are temporary, because the protein eventually dissolves, so it may be necessary to repeat the procedure six months to several years later, depending on the body chemistry of the individual and on the form of collagen used. Generally, Zyplast® lasts longer than Zyderm®. Long-lasting results also depend on factors such as stress at the treatment site. For instance, laughing, crying, smoking, and enduring sun exposure will speed up rewrinkling! Anyone undergoing this treatment must recognize that the collagen injections will not last forever; and protection from the sun is essential.

Fat Injections

The idea of transferring fat from one part of the body to another in order to correct various defects is not new, but the procedure was rarely performed until the introduction of fat suctioning. Fat suctioning or liposuction may be familiar to you as a way of getting rid of unwanted fat that causes bulged, diet-and-exercise-doesn't-help-much hips, buttocks, and thighs. In liposuction, incisions are made into an area where there is an excess of this fat, and it is suctioned out by a high-pressure vacuum system.

For the purpose of reducing or eliminating facial wrinkles, fat tissue is obtained in semiliquid form from an area adjacent to the stomach;

this tissue is then injected into the wrinkled area of the face. The relatively simple procedure involved was first introduced in the mid-1980s, but the jury is still out on whether it is successful. At question are the viability of the fat that is removed and the length of time before the wrinkles return. Because they constitute an autologous procedure—a procedure in which something is taken from the body and then reintroduced to it—fat injections do not fit the definition of a product or a medication, and therefore they do not require FDA approval.

Fibril Injections

Fibril is a synthetic substance that offers a new alternative to collagen and fat injections. Researchers who have been studying fibril gel since 1984 say that it may be a very effective treatment for patients who are allergic to collagen. It is thought that fibril may stimulate the production of replacement collagen in the injection location. Approved by the FDA in 1988, fibril injections have provided longer-lasting results than collagen in clinical studies. But as with collagen injections, stress at the location of the implant contributes to the wrinkles' return. Since the procedure is still somewhat new, patients considering it should determine whether the physician is experienced with the particular material.

Silicone Injections

You don't hear too much anymore about this method of treating wrinkles, perhaps because it never received FDA approval for that purpose. Silicone is a synthetic plastic that can be injected into the body. When injected into wrinkles or deeper furrows it can smooth them out. Unlike collagen, is is nonallergenic and doesn't have the disadvantage of eventually dissolving. However, it can cause a permanent unsightly bulge, either because the injection wasn't placed perfectly or because it shifted. Sometimes impurities slip into the silicone during the manufacturing process that can cause chronic (and sometimes severe) skin reactions. Additionally, there are no well-recognized standard procedures for ensuring the purity of silicone.

Topical Chemotherapy

Chemotherapy is defined as treatment by means of drugs. It has become most widely known as a treatment for cancer. When an anticancer drug in cream or lotion form is applied to the skin surface, the procedure is described as topical chemotherapy. Precancerous actinic keratoses are successfully treated with the drug fluorouracil, known variously as 5-fluorouracil, 5-FU, Adrucil, Fluoroplex, and Efudex. 5-FU is an antimetabolite cancer drug that is given internally to patients suffering from internal cancers, to inhibit cancer cell growth. These patients often experience gastrointestinal side effects and lowered blood counts. But since only about 6 percent of a dose applied to the skin is absorbed, none of these systemic side effects occurs when 5-FU is used in topical chemotherapy.

For widespread actinic keratoses—especially of the face and scalp—and for some basal cell carcinomas (to be discussed in chapter 14) 5-FU is very successful. It is also safe, easy to administer, and produces excellent cosmetic results: skin often looks smoother and younger. 5-FU can not only eradicate visible precancerous lesions, but actually seek out and destroy those that remain hidden below the surface of the skin. Occasionally, 5-FU is used to treat just a few actinic keratoses, if they are in a place of cosmetic importance. This is because the scarring or change in pigmentation that may result from cryotherapy or electrodesiccation is unlikely to occur with 5-FU.

Topical 5-FU is available from the manufacturer as a solution or cream formulated at different strengths, ranging from 1 to 5 percent. Fairer-skinned people frequently are given lower strengths of the drug. Depending on the type of lesion to be treated and the skin type of the individual, a physician may decide to use a stronger concentration, which can be made up by a pharmacist.

The patient usually applies the 5-FU sparingly and carefully twice daily to the affected areas of skin, using the fingertips and carefully avoiding the eyes, nose, and mouth. The use of cosmetics or other creams during treatment is usually discouraged. The sun must be avoided, too, because it can greatly intensify the expected inflammatory response. Tretinoin (Retin-A®) is sometimes added to enhance the penetration of 5-FU. Patients are seen regularly by the physician, who will decide whether treatment should be discontinued or changed in some way.

By the end of the second week or early in the third week, the skin begins to look dreadful! It is red and dry and may be accompanied by blisters, oozing, and discomfort such as might be encountered after sunburn. Occasionally, an allergic reaction or severe irritation may arise soon after treatment is begun. This usually responds to anti-inflammatory corticosteroid creams; painkillers may be used if necessary. The inflammation usually affects only areas where there are lesions, leaving the adjacent skin unaffected.

Usually the patient applies the 5-FU for 3 to 4 weeks. At the end of that time, if all of the keratoses have not disappeared or been destroyed, another treatment regimen of 5-FU may be recommended.

Actinic keratoses on the scalp, neck, back, chest, and backs of the hands usually require longer treatment than those on the face. Healing begins to take place as soon as the treatment is discontinued, and within a few weeks the skin looks far better than it did before treatment began. At times, 5-FU may be combined with other chemicals to eradicate various lesions associated with photodamage. 5-FU does not prevent the development of new keratoses in the future.

Tretinoin (Trade Name: Retin-A®)

By now most people have heard of Retin-A®. It's the so-called fountain-of-youth drug that can actually make wrinkles disappear. Unlike various high-priced cosmetics that have been touted to do this but never really smoothed anything out but your wallet, tretinoin has been proved to reduce fine wrinkling, pore size, and mottled pigmentation; it can also stimulate blood flow to give a youthful rosy glow to the skin. Clinical evidence shows that it increases collagen formation and skin cell turnover, resulting in a thicker epidermis and distributing melanin pigment evenly throughout the epidermis. At the same time, the stratum corneum (the lowest layer of skin) is thinned, which helps rough, sun-damaged skin become smoother and younger looking. Tretinoin can fade solar lentigines and telangiectasia and can even reduce actinic keratoses.

This doesn't happen overnight, of course, but after four to six months of regular use, people look as if they have had a dermabrasion or chemical peel. It's not a substitute for a face-lift for sagging skin, but it is an effective way to turn back the clock just a bit and to improve photoaged skin. Although many people who have used tretinoin are very pleased with it, others have been disappointed. They could not or would not tolerate some of the irritating effects of the treatment that may occur such as dryness, peeling, redness, and swelling. Nevertheless, individuals who stay with the initial treatment plan for eight to twelve months, followed by a maintenance schedule, are usually very satisfied with the results.

Clinical Studies of Tretinoin

Retin-A® has an interesting history. Tretinoin (all-trans-retinoic), a vitamin A derivative, was first synthesized chemically in 1946. Approved by the FDA in 1971 for the treatment of common acne, it has been available by prescription in various concentrations in cream, gell, and liquid formulations.

Albert M. Kligman, MD, emeritus professor of dermatology at the University of Pennsylvania School of Medicine and the universally acknowledged pioneer in treating acne with tretinoin, says that for years patients told him that after a few months of successful treatment for their acne their skin was smoother, its texture was better, and some of the blotches were fading. "I thought these were just enthusiastic patients," said Dr. Kligman. But finally Dr. Kligman and his associates decided to do a small double-blind study (where neither the physicians nor the patients know which individuals are getting a specific active treatment and which are getting applications of something inert); and he says, "We found that their enthusiasm was justified, because they were right."

Although Dr. Kligman discovered tretinoin's usefulness in treating sun-damaged skin, another group of researchers provided the first proof of its efficacy in treating the problem. Led by John J. Voorhees, MD, professor and chairman of dermatology at the University of Michigan Medical School, the group published its study in the prestigious *Journal of the American Medical Association* in January of 1988. Dr. Voorhees said, "All patients continued to show some improvement in the condition of their skin during the study. Of course, some patients showed greater improvement than others, but the fact is the amount of wrinkling, roughness, and age spots was reduced by a greater or lesser degree in each patient.

"With tretinoin," Dr. Voorhees explained, "new skin cells push toward the surface and this clears the skin of dead cells and other debris. There is a fading of age spots and a stimulation of collagen production. At the same time there is an increase in the amount of blood circulating to the skin, and the skin has a healthier appearance. Cell growth becomes more even."

Another interesting study used computerized measurements of silicone impressions from wrinkled skin to prove that tretinoin is effective in reducing wrinkles. James J. Leyden, MD, professor of dermatology at the University of Pennsylvania School of Medicine, remarks, "The system shows that tretinoin does work. It takes some of the subjectivity out of evaluation and gives us, for the first time, an objective method of measuring the drug's effect." He continues, "This is much more accurate than relying solely on a patient's or physician's evaluation. It's even better than photographs, because of the difficulty in duplicating lighting conditions from time to time."

How true. We all look better from time to time, depending on the lighting in a room, on whether we've had a good rest the night before, and—as I laughingly said at my recent high-school class reunion—on whether our friends are wearing their glasses! A study that objectively demonstrates that tretinoin works to reduce wrinkling is therefore very convincing. However, some physicians are less enthusiastic about it, citing patients' complaints that the irritating effects of the drug reduce its appeal for them.

Other Uses of Tretinoin

Tretinoin also shows promise as a treatment for some forms of cancer—particularly in preventing the progression of premalignant growths, such as actinic keratoses, into skin cancer.

Barbara A. Gilchrest, MD, professor and chairman of dermatology at Boston University School of Medicine, says that dramatic improvements from applications of tretinoin are being shown in initial reports from a study done at ten centers. Each patient in the study applied the tretinoin topically to actinic keratoses. Researchers report that the number and size of lesions dropped during treatment with the drug. "Tretinoin has enormous potential implications for treating other age-associated medical conditions," Dr. Gilchrest said.

FDA Approval Sought

But at this point, the manufacturer of Retin-A® is only claiming that it is effective in treating acne; as yet the manufacturer has not received FDA approval for other claims. Ortho, a subsidiary of Johnson & Johnson and the manufacturer of Retin-A®, submitted a new drug application to the Food and Drug Administration (FDA) in July of 1989. The application is for tretinoin cream in a 0.05 strength. The inactive ingredients in it differ slightly from those in the Retin-A® that has been approved for treating acne. Ortho plans to give the tretinoin a new brand name, when and if it gets FDA approval. To gain FDA approval, a drug must be evaluated and approved for safety and for effectiveness in treating what it is supposed to treat. Thus, Ortho must prove that its tretinoin is both safe to use and effective in reducing sun-caused wrinkles. The length of time from when a new drug application is submitted until an opinion is handed down by the

FDA averages about 30 months, so Ortho is unlikely to get approval before 1991. The application included a summary of the results of a randomized 650-person double-blind study conducted at nine different sites across the country.

Even before FDA approval was sought, physicians everywhere began prescribing it for patients. That's because a physician can, at his or her discretion, prescribe a drug to be used for some purpose other than that for which the drug company has received FDA approval to market it. Another good example of this situation involves minoxidil, a drug approved for treatment of hypertension; in the early to middle 1980s, minoxidil showed promise of spurring growth of hair in some balding men. For several years before Upjohn, the manufacturer, received FDA approval to market the drug for this purpose, doctors were prescribing it for patients. Interestingly, some studies suggest that Retin-A® may increase the effectiveness of minoxidil, (now known as Rogaine®) for hair growth.

All of this means that many dermatologists are already recommending and prescribing tretinoin to their patients for the purpose of reducing wrinkles. If, after consulting with a dermatologist who is experienced in using it, you elect to undergo treatment, you should expect to have the following experiences.

How Tretinoin Is Used

You will give yourself the treatment every day, every other day, or every third day, depending on your skin type and your doctor's recommendation. Generally, people whose complexion is fair, who have a history of skin sensitivity, or who are elderly are advised either to use a lower concentration of tretinoin or to use it with less frequency. About 20 to 30 minutes before bedtime, you will wash the treatment area with a mild, nonirritating soap, gently lathering it with your fingertips or with a soft washcloth. Then you will rinse the skin carefully. After the skin is completely dry, you will apply the tretinoin sparingly to the photodamaged skin—face, scalp, hands, forearms, and V of the neck. Using a pea-sized amount of the cream, you apply it with your fingertips, spreading it evenly over your entire face. If you have very oily skin, your doctor may recommend that you use the gel formulation, which is more irritating than the cream. You can go close to your eyes with the medication but not actually *in* them. Your doctor probably will caution you not to use it on your upper eye lid, either. In addition, most doctors recommend that you not place the medication in the corners of your nose or at the angles of your mouth.

If you wear eyeglasses, don't put them on after the treatment; if they were to rest on the bridge of the nose or even touch your face, occlusion would occur, heightening the risk of irritation in the area. Eyeglasses might also spread the medication into your eyes. You will also be discouraged from exercising or in any other way exposing yourself to excessive heat or perspiration just after the tretinoin has been applied. For this reason, application before bedtime is best for most people. Five minutes after applying it, you should apply a water-based moisturizer.

It is unwise to use exfolients, abrasive scrubs, toners, astringents, or any lotions or skin fresheners containing high concentrations of alcohol during this therapy. Avoid weather extremes, such as heat, stiff wind, or cold. A moisturizer worn during the day is useful in alleviating any tight, dry feelings that arise from the treatment. If (as occasionally happens) your skin becomes very red or severely in-flamed, your doctor may prescribe a steroid cream or ointment to control it.

Tretinoin-treated Skin Is Super-sensitive to the Sun

Because anyone undergoing tretinoin treatment becomes extremely sensitive to the sun, a sunscreen is an absolute necessity! If you opt for this treatment, do everything you can to minimize your sun exposure, as described in Part Two. Women may find it useful on a general year-round basis to use a moisturizer with an SPF of 15 under or in place of makeup; alternatively, they may prefer to use an emollient sunscreen. Men can use a sunscreen as an after-shave lotion. Sunscreens that have an SPF higher than 15 are usually unnecessary and may indeed have too high a concentration of potentially irritating chemicals. If you get sunburned despite your best intentions, your doctor will probably tell you to discontinue the treatment temporarily. Likewise, your doctor may recommend that you suspend treatment if you are going to be vacationing in a sunny climate or taking a ski trip.

Tretinoin and Effects on Babies

Tretinoin is chemically related to isotretinoin (also known as 13-cis-retinoic acid or Acutane®), an orally administered drug used for treatment of acne. Isotretinoin has raised concern about the safety of Retin-A® because it has been associated with birth defects when used by pregnant women. Although there is no indication that topical use of tretinoin has the same effects, systemic absorption, especially through inflamed skin (a frequent effect of the medication) is a possibility. Thus, most physicians discourage women from undergoing topical tretinoin treatment while planning to become pregnant, actually being pregnant, or nursing.

Is it wise to let a baby or young child come in contact with your skin if you are using tretinoin? I've been giving serious thought to using topical tretinoin, and since one of the great pleasures in my life is to hug and kiss my grandchildren, I posed this question to Dr. Albert Lefkovits, of the Mount Sinai School of Medicine. He said, "Since you apply the medicine before going to sleep, if you wash your face in the morning, there should be no residue on the skin when you see the children."

Tretinoin and Cancer

According to the Skin Cancer Foundation, a number of people have begun to think of topical tretinoin as an anticancer agent. It may have gotten that reputation because it makes some actinic keratoses disappear, but it has not been proved to be effective in preventing new ones from developing. In one study, some early actinic keratoses improved, but most advanced ones didn't improve much, and some actually progressed to invasive squamous cell carcinomas during treatment. Nonetheless, many physicians recommend using oral tretinoin for extensive actinic keratoses, much as they would prescribe 5-FU.

There have also been some reports that tretinoin, together with sunlight, could increase the incidence of skin cancer. Indeed, studies done on hairless, albino mice indicated this. Studies on humans show that topical tretinoin decreases the adhesion of keratin cells on the outer layer of the skin, which makes the skin look younger but at the same time reduces the protection offered by those tougher skin cells, thus making the skin more sensitive. So if you decide to use tretinoin to counter the effects of years of sun exposure, be aware that this is not a license to start all over again to be incautious in the sun. The steps to younger, less-wrinkled skin are simple: consider a program of tretinoin treatments, and protect yourself from further sun exposure.

A Drug, Not a Cosmetic

Unfortunately, many people are using tretinoin without medical supervision. A word of advice here: never use someone else's prescription, for this or any other drug. It may not be the right strength for you—the directions for you may be different than for a friend—and if the drug is obtained through some roundabout means (out of country, a laboratory with indiscriminate standards, or the like), proper control may not have been maintained over the product. Tretinoin is a drug, not a cosmetic. You need a physician's guidance when using it.

You may have noticed some cosmetics with names that sound similar to tretinoin or Retin-A®. Although retinol is a form of vitamin A, it has never been demonstrated to work in the same way as Retin-A®. Keep in mind that, without FDA approval, cosmetic companies are prohibited from claiming that their product can change the structure of the skin (and thus get rid of wrinkles). As of mid-1990, no cosmetic or drug (including tretinoin) has obtained that approval.

More Than One Treatment may be Indicated

There are several ways to treat sun-damaged skin, and combinations of treatments are often successful. For instance, face-lifts may be combined with topical tretinoin treatments.

If you are considering a treatment strictly for cosmetic purposes, you may wish to meet with a dermatologist and a plastic surgeon, and even get a second or third opinion. Listen carefully to the options outlined for you, and then decide if you want to choose one of them. Such treatment is considered elective—meaning that it's not urgent—and it is really up to you!

If you have a precancerous condition such as actinic keratoses or nevi, heed the advice of a dermatologist, perhaps getting a second opinion. But don't reject treatment altogether, since some treatment, while usually not urgent, is ultimately necessary. Waiting too long can mean developing cancer and having to undergo far more extensive treatment than would have been required if you had begun it earlier.

Is Treatment Expensive?

Private physicians' fees vary from one community to another, but most physicians are willing to adjust fees or to work out a special schedule of payments with you. Insurance companies that pay or reimburse in part or in whole for treatment of medical conditions may not pay for strictly cosmetic treatments. But sometimes they will pay or reimburse if scarring or serious photodamage has significantly affected your self-image and self-esteem. Treatment is often available on a sliding fee scale at a local hospital that has a clinic or is involved in research.

Is Treatment Necessary?

If you have developed precancerous actinic keratoses or dysplastic nevi, it is important that you be evaluated by a dermatologist. But if you have thus far only developed wrinkles as the result of photodamage, you may choose not to do anything to reduce or reverse them. But, please, protect yourself from the sun now to avoid any greater cumulative damage, which might lead to skin cancer. And remember that evidence now exists that sun protection can not only stop ongoing damage but also allow some natural regeneration (read: rejuvenation) to occur.

Wrinkles aren't so bad: the wonderful actress, Helen Hayes, likes to refer to them as her "service stripes." A favorite child I know once said, "I like people with crinkly skin. They like to read stories and buy presents, and they let you stay up late."

If you don't want to try tretinoin, but you're dissatisfied with your photoaged skin, remember that a sunny disposition and becoming clothes and hairstyle can go a long way toward making you an attractive person. There are also a number of excellent ways to camouflage discolorations and other cosmetic defects.

Camouflage

Pigmentation problems, scars from treatments, telangiectasia (a condition characterized by prominent blood vessels), and various sun-induced damage cannot always be successfully reversed. In addition, some procedures to correct problems may themselves result in unsightly pigmentation problems or scars. Thus, additional surgery or treatment may not be the answer.

At one time, various nonprescription bleach products containing amoniated mercury were popular, although they were not very effective. Unfortunately, they caused many allergic reactions and could be absorbed by the body, causing other adverse reactions. Consequently, these products were banned by the FDA in 1974. Today, some lightening agents containing the safer hydroquinone are available; but they, too, are often ineffective, and they can cause irritation that may increase pigmentation or cause complete loss of it.

Fortunately, marvelous products are made that disguise even the most unsightly scars. A number of companies (such as Dermablend) make long-lasting, greaseless, waterproof concealers that offer good coverage and match or blend into any color of skin—from the palest Celtic to the darkest African. Generally these products do not contain perfumes or irritating ingredients, and they can be worn without any makeup or under your usual makeup. If they aren't available at your local pharmacy or department store, ask your dermatologist for advice and suggestions. For a nearby location that sells Dermablend, you can write to Dermablend Corrective Cosmetics, P. O. Box 601, Farmingdale, New Jersey 07727.

Summary

The sun has a powerful effect on the skin. Heatstroke is a medical emergency; sunburn usually responds to home remedies. Cumulative damage from the sun is treatable and often reversible. Dermatologists and sometimes plastic surgeons can offer a number of therapeutic options.

Dermabrasion (a form of skin planing) and chemical peels can remove many sun-caused imperfections, as well as other scars, leaving you with a "new" skin. Cryosurgery, which makes use of freezing chemicals to remove many small growths, is another option. Surgery may use electric power or the traditional scalpel to rid the body of unwanted growths. Collagen, fat, silicone, or fibril injections can fill depressions in the face formed by scarring or sun-induced wrinkles. Topical chemotherapy (5-FU) removes actinic keratoses, the precancerous lesions caused by the sun.

Tretinoin (Retin-A®), heralded as the fountain-of-youth drug, successfully treats photodamaged skin and reduces wrinkles. Most clinical studies give it high marks, and patients too have been clamoring for it. It is especially important for individuals who use it to take precautions to avoid exposure to the sun. Tretinoin is sometimes available to people without medical supervision, but it is very unwise to administer it without medical guidance: it is a drug, not a cosmetic. No over-the-counter drug or cosmetic has been demonstrated to reduce wrinkles, but the makers of a particular formulation of tretinoin may get FDA approval for their product in the early 1990s.

Insurance will pay for some treatments for sun-damaged skin. And clinics will adjust fees to make it available to those who need or want it.

High-quality blemish concealers are available and should be considered by anyone who wants to hide unattractive growths, scars, or irregular pigmentation.

14 Treating Cancer of the Skin: Basal Cell Carcinoma, Squamous Cell Carcinoma, and Melanoma

The word cancer often evokes frightening thoughts and feelings. And no wonder: cancer is characterized by abnormal cell growth, is capable of spreading through the body, and is often life-threatening.

Cancer is actually a group of different diseases that share some common features: the cells are irregular and disordered, and they serve no useful function. Unlike normal cells that wear out and die, malignant (cancerous) cells continue to divide and multiply, reproducing themselves and invading and destroying surrounding tissues.

Cancer of the skin acts the same way, and although highly treatable, it can be serious. As we discussed in chapter 7, basal cell carcinoma (BCC), the most common of all skin cancers, is most often found on the face, scalp, or neck, and sometimes on the trunk. It grows slowly and is almost always curable by one or more of the treatments to be described in this chapter. Although BCC may recur in the same place or somewhere else, it will again respond to prompt treatment. If it is ignored and neglected until it has grown large and penetrated through other layers of skin, however, it becomes more difficult to cure and may result in cosmetically unacceptable scarring.

Squamous cell carcinoma (SCC), the second most common type of skin cancer, grows faster than BCC, can invade and destroy underlying tissues, and can also metastasize (spread) to lymph nodes or glands or to other parts of the body.

SCC often arises on sun-exposed areas of the body such as the top of the nose or ears and the backs of the hands, or in areas that have been subjected to X-ray treatment, scars, and ulcerations. Metastasis is more likely to occur in those lesions that appear on areas of the body not exposed to the sun. Squamous cell carcinomas are generally removed by one of several types of surgery, possibly followed by radiation therapy. If the cancer has spread, a combination of treatments is often used.

Other skin cancers (whether sun-related or not) such as Bowen's disease, keratoacanthoma, and xeroderma pigmetosa are treated in much the same way as are basal cell carcinoma and squamous cell carcinoma.

As detailed in chapter 8, melanoma is a life-threatening form of cancer that usually begins on an existing mole or develops in a new one and can spread throughout the body. It is likely to arise on the back, face, or lower legs in women and on the torso of men, but it can begin anywhere on the body.

The size or type of growth, its location on the body, whether it has already metastasized, and the age and general medical condition of the patient all help determine the best method of treatment. When any of several treatments would be appropriate, the patient and physician together may choose one based on personal preference. Most procedures for skin cancer are performed either in a physician's office or in the outpatient department of a hospital.

Regardless of which treatment you undergo, recovery is usually free of complications. Before departing from the treatment room, you may get instructions such as the following:

* Avoid disturbing the wound or scar; wash and dry the area gently.
* Take an antibiotic orally, or apply it in ointment form to the treated area.
* If needed, take a mild analgesic for pain.
* Report any pain, swelling, drainage, or increased bleeding, unless specifically told to expect it.
* Call the physician if you develop any signs of infection, such as headache, muscle aches, dizziness, or a general flulike feeling or fever.

In subsequent pages, we will review various treatments; some of these may be included with a biopsy, while others may follow it.

Surgery

Surgery is the practice of treating diseases, injuries, and deformities by operation, using manipulation or instruments. The removal of a growth or lesion on the skin for medical or cosmetic reasons, by any means, is considered dermatological surgery. As discussed in detail in chapter 13, three standard types relevant to skin cancer are excisional surgery, electrosurgery, and cryosurgery. Other types (to be discussed separately later in this chapter) are laser surgery and chemosurgery (Mohs surgery).

Topical Chemotherapy: 5-FU

Although most cancerous lesions, regardless of size, can be surgically removed, other modalities are often just as successful and may place less stress on a patient. Topical chemotherapy is such a modality. Treatment of actinic keratoses—especially when they are widespread—frequently makes use of topical chemotherapy. It is often used for basal cell carcinomas and squamous cell carcinomas, as well as for the precancerous lesions. 5-FU is described in full in chapter 13.

Radiation Therapy

The use of high-energy radiation in the treatment of disease, especially cancer, was first introduced early in this century. Also known as *radiotherapy* or *X-ray therapy*, it involves directing beams at malignant cells, damaging and often killing them. Treatment is planned and supervised by a radiotherapist or radiation oncologist—a physician who is a specialist in radiation therapy for cancer—often in consultation with the dermatologist who initially diagnosed the skin cancer. Radiotherapy can be administered in an outpatient department of a hospital or in a radiotherapist's office.

Skin cancers that are difficult to remove surgically, such as those occurring on the tip of the nose and at the top of the ear, may be treated with radiotherapy. The invisible rays can also damage normal, healthy cells, but these recover; still, care is taken to protect the normal skin. Treatment is generally scheduled over a period of time, often several sessions within a few weeks; but if a tumor is less than 1 cm in diameter, one dose may be sufficient.

Laser Surgery

The term *laser* is an acronym for Light Amplification by Stimulated Emission of Radiation. Laser beams are an extremely concentrated source of light, and they give off so much heat that they destroy anything in their path. Thousands of times more intense than the most powerful light beams, they can be narrowed and aimed so accurately at cancerous cells and delivered so speedily that they destroy only the diseased tissue, without affecting the surrounding healthy areas. The laser is a "no-touch" technique that sterilizes as it works. A significant feature of laser surgery is that it coagulates (clots) blood, thus controlling bleeding. It is useful for treating various skin cancers.

Several different types of lasers are in dermatologic use today, and many physicians are especially trained in the technique. They may be members of the American Board of Laser Surgery as well as members of the board of their original specialty.

Chemosurgery (Mohs Surgery)

In the early 1940s, Dr. Frederic Mohs, a professor of surgery at the University of Michigan, developed a technique of microscopically controlled surgery called *chemosurgery*. As originally conceived, a strong chemical such as zinc chloride may be applied to certain skin cancers and left there for up to 24 hours, during which time it kills the cancerous cells. The cells are then removed and examined under a microscope. The procedure can be repeated until all cancer cells have been removed. When all the tissue seen under the microscope is normal, the operating physician concludes that enough has been removed. This procedure is known as a *fixed-tissue* technique.

The *fresh-tissue* technique is a similar but newer procedure that is more commonly used today. The chemical paste is omitted, and the suspected area is cut out and examined microscopically. The procedure is repeated as often as necessary until the lesion is completely eradicated. This method preserves more normal tissue than the usual excisional surgery, especially when the margin between healthy and cancerous tissue is not clearly defined. Frequently the tumor (basal cell carcinoma, squamous cell carcinoma, melanoma, or some other skin cancer) can be removed in a single office or clinic visit. Sometimes hospitalization is necessary.

The procedure, now most commonly called *Mohs surgery,* is indicated for the following types of lesions:

★ Large (greater than 2 cm in diameter)

★ Not completely removed previously
★ Present for a long time
★ Possessing an indistinct margin between cancerous and healthy skin
★ Recurrent (initially removed, but grew back)
★ Located in areas that have high recurrence rates (such as on or around the ear, at the fold between the mouth and nose, on the nose itself, on or in the nostrils, on the scalp, or at the center of the face)
★ On young people, because these are likely to recur
★ Located in areas where it is vital to save as much of the normal tissue as possible (such as on the penis, the nose, the lips, a finger, an eyelid, or an ear)
★ Certain basal cell carcinomas known as *morpheaform BCC* (characterized by a thickened, unusually fibrous growth)

Mohs surgery is a highly specialized procedure that requires considerable training and experience; not all dermatologists perform it. If your doctor suspects or has determined by biopsy that a lesion is cancerous, and if he or she feels that this procedure would be the appropriate way to treat it, you may be referred to a Mohs surgery specialist. If you think that your lesion fits some of the preceding criteria, you should feel comfortable in bringing up the subject of Mohs surgery, even if your dermatologist doesn't suggest it.

Prior to beginning the procedure, the physician will treat the area of the skin that is to undergo the surgery with an anesthetic. Most of the visible cancer is then scraped away with a curette, and a thin piece of tissue beneath and around the scraped skin is surgically removed. The excised tissue is divided into pieces, which are rapidly frozen and then examined under a microscope while the patient waits in the office or clinic. If the doctor determines that no cancer cells are present in the frozen tissue, no additional surgery is performed, and the patient can prepare to leave. But if cancer cells remain, another layer of tissue is surgically removed, frozen, and examined under the microscope. The procedure is repeated until no cancer cells remain in either the base or the sides of the area where the visible tumor was scraped away.

Patients who undergo this procedure may need to have two, three, or four layers of tissue (called *stages*) removed before the surgery is completed. Each surgical process takes 20 to 30 minutes, but time expended on the preparation of slides and on the physician's interpretation of them adds to the total. Thus, a patient may have to spend an entire day at the doctor's office or clinic.

After the surgery is completed, the patient goes home. The surgeon usually gives the patient careful instructions for self-care at home, as well as advice about when to call the doctor. Mild analgesics are usually sufficient to counteract pain. Any bleeding can be controlled by applying pressure with a sterile gauze pad. Some swelling, bruising, or redness may occur, but that usually subsides within a few days. Infections occur occasionally.

The wound that results from Mohs surgery may heal by itself in 4 to 8 weeks, in a process called *spontaneous granulation,* or it may be closed with sutures (stitches). Because the wound will drain, a clean dressing must be kept on it, changed daily by the patient. In some situations where the destruction from the chemosurgery is disfiguring, reconstructive procedures may be indicated.

Many physicians are trained in this technique. Perry Robbins, MD, is internationally recognized as a Mohs surgery specialist, and he has trained many of these doctors. He is chief of the Mohs surgery unit at the New York University Medical Center and is the founder and president of the Skin Cancer Foundation. In a pamphlet he gives his patients, Dr. Robbins writes, "Experience has shown that, if there is a recurrence, it will usually be within the first year following surgery." Dr. Robbins, like other Mohs surgeons, tells his patients to see their dermatologists regularly for at least five years following such surgery; he strongly recommends that, if they notice anything unusual on their skin, they call the doctor's attention to it.

Mohs surgery is the procedure of choice for combating many skin cancers. It is usually not indicated for those that are small, can easily be removed by other methods, or have a distinct margin between themselves and the normal skin.

Immunotherapy

Although it is not used as the initial or primary treatment for skin cancer, immunotherapy has a definite role in the treatment of individuals who have multiple extensive superficial skin cancers or multiple premalignant skin lesions. Immunotherapy attempts to stimulate and strengthen the body's own natural defenses for protection against and recovery from disease.

As was discussed in chapter 2, there are three major forms of immunological activity in the body:

★ *Antibody response* is produced by B cells, which are manufactured in the bone marrow. These cells produce antibodies that help defend the body against infection or toxic substances.

★ *Cellular immune response* is produced by lymphocytes (or T cells), which mature in the thymus gland and are stimulated by antigens to circulate through the body.

★ *Natural killer (NK) cells* are stimulated by viral infections, possibly through production of interferon—a chemical substance that is naturally released by the body in response to viral infections. This natural resistance differs from the immunity acquired as a result of previous exposure and is not caused by B or T cells.

It is now widely recognized that individuals with a suppressed or deficient immune system are vulnerable and prone to many diseases, including cancer. It is also recognized that cancer patients are susceptible to infections and other illnesses, because their immunity is low. Studies mentioned in chapter 2 have demonstrated that exposure to ultraviolet radiation can lower the immune system.

Theoretically, improving and repairing the immune system of a cancer patient should lead to greater control and eventually the cure of the disease, and indeed this often occurs. Consequently researchers continue to develop and test various vaccines and other products that are designed to help the body help itself, by persuading the immune system to recognize and reject cancer cells. Immunological methods may be recommended as a treatment for skin cancer patients, usually after the original tumor or lesion has been destroyed by surgery, radiation, or topical chemotherapy. Often the chemicals used in immunotherapy are injected under the skin or into a vein so that they circulate throughout the body; alternatively they may be injected directly into the tumor or taken by mouth. Chemicals such as dinitrochlorobenzene (DNCB) cream may be applied to the skin repeatedly, resulting in the disappearance of the cancer.

Tumor-specific antigens are produced by collecting cancer cells from the patient growing them in a laboratory culture, and then treating the cultured cells with various chemicals to uncover the antigens. These treated cancer cells are injected back into the patient in the hope that, like a vaccination, they will produce an immune response to the tumor.

Interferon, a substance named for its ability to interfere with viral infections, is released naturally by animals and humans as a response to invading viruses. In some instances, interferon recognizes, suppresses, and destroys cancer cells, and it can trigger the immune system. When first harnessed for use with cancer patients, it was in very short supply; but it has now been synthesized in the laboratory and is used in combination with chemotherapy for internal cancers, including melanoma. It may be applied to a lesion in the form of an ointment, or it may be injected directly into the lesion.

Treatments of the sort just described are not routine. They are most likely to be offered to people who have experienced a recurrence or metastasis of their cancer. Immunotherapy, when it involves the circulation of therapeutic drugs or antigens throughout the body, may produce some side effects, such as tiredness, fever, inflammation, or mild pain around the site of the treatment. Occasionally, chills or lymph node swelling may occur.

Combination Treatments for BCC and SCC

A combination of the preceding therapies may be used for any particular skin cancer. For instance, a tumor or lesion may be surgically excised, and then the base may be frozen with liquid nitrogen. Excision permits the upper level and margins to be sent for pathological examination, which the cryosurgery allows for a more complete cleanup. After surgery has been performed, radiation may be advised; and Mohs surgery may be indicated for a lesion that wasn't fully removed at all the margins during a previous phase of the treatment.

Treatment of Metastatic Squamous Cell Carcinoma

When squamous cell carcinoma invades underlying tissue or structures, it can still be treated in the various ways that have been described already. However, when squamous cell carcinoma acts very aggressively or has been neglected for a long period of time, it can spread to other parts of the body, often through the lymph system. Isolated areas of spread may respond well to radiation therapy, but often when the cancer has metastasized widely it needs to be treated with chemotherapy. Chemotherapy—treating cancer by administering combinations of different chemical substances—works internally and invisibly throughout the body. It is sometimes difficult to understand how it works, but it does. Squamous cell carcinoma responds best to a combination of different drugs; cis-platinum has been particularly successful in treating the disease. Chemotherapy is also used to combat metastatic malignant melanoma and will be discussed more fully later in this chapter.

Individuals faced with any kind of metastatic cancer are best served medically if their treatment plan is the product of consultation among specialists working as a team. A medical oncologist (a physician who specializes in the medical treatment of cancer) is likely to lead the team, but radiation oncologists will certainly be consulted, too. If the cancer originated in the skin (as with squamous cell carcinoma), the dermatologist will be an important member of the team and a general or plastic surgeon may also assume an important role. Patients with metastatic squamous cell carcinoma can be optimistic about the outcome of their treatment, because their prognosis is very good.

Follow-up Treatment for BCC and SCC

If you have had a basal cell carcinoma or a squamous cell carcinoma, you are at great risk of developing another. For this reason, your doctor will urge you to examine yourself regularly for any new growths and to schedule regular follow-up visits. And quite naturally you will be urged to lessen the chance of recurrence by protecting yourself from the sun—avoiding it whenever possible, wearing protective clothing, and using sunscreen with an SPF of 15 or more.

Checking for Melanoma

As you know from our previous discussions, malignant melanoma is a cancer that usually begins in a pigmented mole. One of the various surgical methods described previously may be used to remove the primary tumor, along with surrounding tissue, and then a biopsy is performed on it. If the melanoma is detected early, most patients are cured by this method. If the melanoma proves to be malignant, other diagnostic tests must be performed to determine whether the disease has spread beyond its original site.

Has Melanoma Metastasized?

When melanoma is initially diagnosed, it may already have spread, or this may occur later. Such metastasis may occur on the skin itself, beneath it, or in the lymph nodes. Other common sites of metastatic disease include the lungs, the liver, the bone, the gastrointestinal tract, and the central nervous system. In addition, malignant melanoma can spread to such organs as the kidneys, the adrenal glands, and the spleen. Many of the tests that help determine whether the cancer has metastasized—including X-rays, nuclear scans, and ultrasound—come under the general term of *body imaging*. Contrast dye may be swallowed or injected into the body before the picture is taken. Body imaging is performed in a radiologist's office or in the radiology or nuclear medicine department of a hospital. A radiologist is a physician who specializes in various kinds of body imaging, many of which make use of radioactive substances. A specialist in nuclear medicine is trained in several disciplines—among them newer types of nuclear scans that involve the release of small amounts of radionuclides, called *radiopharmaceuticals*, which circulate through tissues, organs, and organ systems (depending on how they are administered) and help highlight these structures for the picture.

Among the body-imaging tests that may be used to determine where and how much melanoma has spread are the following:

* Conventional X-rays
* CAT scans—a technique that makes use of computers and X-rays to obtain a highly detailed image of a section of the body being studied
* Angiograms (also called *arteriograms*), for which dye is introduced into the body so that the vessel structures and arteries leading to various organs are made visible
* Nuclear scans of one or more body parts
* Gallium scans—a nuclear scanning technique that shows rapidly dividing cells and can detect lymph node involvement
* Ultrasound, which produces a picture called a *sonogram* by means of high-frequency sound waves that enable the viewer to examine the position, form, and function of anatomical structures, without resort to radiation or injection of a dye or chemical
* Magnetic Resonance Imaging (MRI)—a noninvasive technique

that, like the CAT scan, produces a three-dimensional, cross-sectional body image, but that uses radio waves and a magnetic field (rather than radiation) to delineate the tissues

After all the tests are completed, the doctor will have a clear idea of the extent or *stage* of the disease. If you are treated by a medical oncologist who is in private practice or is a full-time member of a medical center, the treatment will be individualized, depending on the stage of the disease and various individual factors. What follows in this chapter is an overview of treatment of metastatic malignant melanoma; but if you or someone you care about has just been diagnosed with metastatic melanoma or is currently receiving treatment for this disease, you will find it helpful to read more about cancer treatment. A number of books that focus on this subject are listed in appendix III.

Treatment of Metastatic Melanoma

Generally, the primary tumor is removed by one of the surgical methods described earlier in this chapter. If melanoma has already spread or if it later recurs with a spread, treatment will be offered, and the wise patient will accept it. Whether the objective is to control or cure melanoma that began on the skin, in the eye (intraocular melanoma), or at an unknown and undiscovered primary site, treatments are similar. However, the specific plan is individualized for each patient.

Like squamous cell carcinoma that has spread through the body, metastatic melanoma requires prompt treatment. This may involve surgical removal of some tumors or clusters of cells, radiation treatment of specific areas of metastasis such as the brain or bones, or chemotherapy for widespread or distant disease (particularly if the lungs or liver are affected). Immunotherapy, which may be combined with chemotherapy or other treatments, is also effective. Any or all of these treatments may be recommended sequentially or in combination.

Surgery for Melanoma

Surgical removal of a melanoma (suspected or positively identified) should be done by a physician experienced in cancer surgery—either a dermatologist or general surgeon. If the melanoma has spread and further surgery is warranted, a general surgeon who specializes in or is experienced in cancer surgery will perform the operation. Lymph nodes are often affected and may have to be removed. This procedure is often referred to as *lymph node dissection,* because the structures are separated along natural lines by cutting or tearing the connective tissue framework, instead of by making a wide incision. When a surgical incision is very large or deep, or is in a particularly exposed area such as the face or neck, replacement skin may have to be grafted from another part of the body. If surgery to repair potential or actual scars is required or desired, it is most often done by a plastic surgeon.

Radiation

Melanoma has often been termed *radioresistant,* meaning that it does not respond well to radiation; consequently, this is not the treatment of choice for controlling or curing the disease. However, it is effective for isolated areas or for palliation—treatment that is not aimed at achieving a cure but at making a patient feel better by relieving symptoms, pain, or discomfort. Radiation is especially useful in providing relief to melanoma patients who have pain in soft tissues or bones, and in improving neurological symptoms that may result from metastasis to the brain.

Chemotherapy

Chemotherapy can reach malignant cells in the body that surgery cannot reach, and others that may have broken away from the original tumor but are too small to be seen under the microscope. Scientists know that, even if only a few malignant cells are seen, others may be lurking around invisibly. These unseen cells can cause recurrence of cancer, even when the original tumor is destroyed or removed. By destroying all or most of these tiny colonies of cancer cells, physicians can often prevent or postpone recurrences. For this reason, chemo-therapy treatment immediately following diagnosis and removal of the primary melanoma—rather than after a recurrence has been recognized—can help achieve long-term control or cure of metastatic melanoma. This principle of treatment is used for many other types of cancers, too.

Types of Drugs

Five major types of drugs and over 100 individual drugs are used to treat cancer, and each works in its own way. A number of them have produced good responses in metastatic malignant melanoma patients. Certain drugs are far more effective when used in combination than when administered separately. It is almost impossible for a nonscientist to gain full mastery or understanding of the detailed workings of these different anticancer agents; and curious as it may seem, even scientists don't always know exactly how each drug works. But to put this limitation into perspective, consider this: even though simple aspirin has been around since almost the beginning of the twentieth century, its precise mechanism still isn't fully understood.

Following are the major categories of anticancer drugs, together with specific examples of drugs from each category that are used to treat metastatic malignant melanoma:

* *Alkylating agents* cause a direct chemical interaction with the cells, blocking their multiplication. Examples include Cisplatin, Carmustine (BCNU), Dacarbazine (DTIC)—an atypical alkylating agent—and Melphalan (L'Pam).
* *Antimetabolites* are "fraudulent nutrients" that cancer cells absorb, at which point the drugs interfere with further growth and replication. An example is Hydroxyurea.
* *Mitotic inhibitors* work to prevent cancer cells from splitting and dividing normally, by interfering with the process needed to produce more cells. An example is Vinblastine.
* *Antitumor antibiotics* interfere with cancer cells' division and growth. They are made from natural substances such as soil fungi. An example is Bleomycin.
* *Hormones* occur naturally in the body, where they function as switches turning on or off the growth or other activity of certain cells in organs. Cancers that depend on hormones for growth can be treated with the opposite hormone (or antihormone). An example is Tamoxifen.

Administration of Drugs

To reach the cancer cells and be effective, medication must enter the bloodstream or pass directly into tumors. Pills taken by mouth in tablet or capsule form are absorbed through the lining of the stomach before entering the bloodstream. Drugs injected into a muscle (intramuscular, or IM injection) eventually enter the bloodstream, too, as do drugs injected directly into the bloodstream through a vein (intravenous, or IV injection). Another way to administer drugs is to drip them slowly into a vein by means of gravity (IV infusion). Alternatively chemotherapy may be introduced directly into a tumor by means of a catheter; this treatment, called *regional perfusion,* is designed to destroy cancer tissue with a minimum of damage to normal surrounding tissue. A catheter is a hollow, flexible tube designed to be passed into a vessel or cavity of the body, where it can then withdraw or inject fluids. Catheters for delivering drugs into the body are inserted in the course of a minor surgical procedure, after which a patient can often go directly home. Sometimes a small pump is implanted into a patient so that a prescribed quantity of chemicals can be released directly into a tumor periodically.

New Drugs

Regardless of where you live, you can obtain the latest FDA-approved drugs, and you may also volunteer for treatment with drugs that are still being studied and tested. This is because physicians throughout the United States and Canada participate in cooperative studies that test new drugs and new ways of using existing drugs. If your own physician cannot tell you about a relevant study of this type, you can contact the Cancer Information Service (CIS) of the National Cancer Institute (NCI) at a toll-free number for more information on how you can join such a study (or as it sometimes called, a *clinical trial*). Information on reaching the NCI is outlined in appendix II.

Activities During Chemotherapy

Many people who receive chemotherapy are able to carry on their usual activities most of the time. Some people find that, for a few days after certain treatments, they just have to take it easy. Others, however, say that the chemotherapy schedule seems to be taking over their lives. If your chemotherapy treatment is really getting you down, consider counseling or join a support or self-help group. Information on finding such help is included in appendix III.

Side Effects

Not everyone has side effects. It is important to differentiate between side effects and symptoms of the disease. Sometimes people who experience adverse side effects misinterpret these as a recurrence or worsening of their disease. Try to maintain an open dialogue with your medical oncologist or with a nurse in the office who can help you sort out some of these concerns.

The side effects of chemotherapy arise because chemotherapy can destroy normal cells as well as cancer cells. The normal cells most likely to be affected are those of the upper gastrointestinal tract, the bone marrow, the hair follicles, and the skin. Chemotherapy drugs can also affect muscles and nerves, and sometimes they cause changes in certain sexual characteristics. Most of the side effects are temporary; but since each person has both a very particular disease and a unique response to treatment (and to the drugs being administered), it is not always easy to predict a patient's reactions.

Following are some side effects that may be experienced, depending on the drugs being taken, the dose, and the individual patient's reactions:

* Fatigue and lack of energy
* Gastrointestinal side effects, including nausea, vomiting, diarrhea, and constipation
* Mouth, gum, and throat dryness or soreness
* Depression of blood cell counts and bone marrow production, resulting in lowered resistance to infection
* Hair loss
* Skin changes, including rashes, itching, or dry, flaky skin
* Muscle and nerve weakness, including tingling or numbing sensations
* Secondary sexual characteristics—a temporary effect of developing "opposite" sexual characteristics if you are taking an antihormone
* Discomfort or pain at the injection site
* Fluid retention, resulting in swelling of the ankles or puffiness of the face

Some of these side effects are also associated with immunotherapy and with other treatments to be described later. Remember, some people have no side effects, while others have many. Most people have just some, and then only at times. If you are having a problem with side effects, your physician or attending nurse can advise you of the many ways to help alleviate these effects; you can also read more about this in the books listed in appendix III.

Perfusion and Hyperthermia

Perfusion for malignant melanoma refers to a procedure in which a very high dose of chemotherapy is administered into an extremity (arm or leg). Hyperthermia is a treatment in which heat is applied to the entire body, to a part of it, or to a tumor only. In a procedure called *isolated perfusion* or *hyperthermia profusion,* the heated area is isolated by means of a tourniquet, and then drugs are administered directly into it. The drugs are flushed out before the tourniquet is released, which allows the chemotherapy to destroy the cancer cells while sparing the patient from adverse side effects of such a large dose of medication. According to many cancer specialists, this type of procedure has often enabled them to avoid amputating an affected limb.

Hyperthermia is sometimes combined with radiation to treat metastases under the skin, yielding better results than radiation alone.

Immunotherapy

Immunotherapy has a definite role in the treatment of metastatic malignant melanoma and has demonstrated effectiveness when administered either directly into the bloodstream or under lesions. Immunotherapy is often combined with chemotherapy; the combination is sometimes called *chemoimmunotherapy.*

You may have heard of interleukin-2, or IL-2, which has recently received much media attention. This substance is formed in small amounts in the body by T cells. When a T cell encounters a foreign antigen, it is activated to produce interleukin-2, which then activates killer cells that merge with the tumor or cancerous cells and kill them. Initially referred to as the *T-cell growth factor* when first identified in 1976, it was later renamed *interleukin-2.* Interleukin is now produced in the laboratory by means of a gene-splicing method. This allows large quantities of the substance to be made, and as a result it is now used in different ways and combinations to treat metastatic malignant melanoma.

Interleukin may be injected directly into the patient for the purpose of enhancing production of white blood cells to attack invading organisms and alien cells, thus boosting the patient's own immune system. It may also be used to treat the patient's own white blood cells after these have been removed; after treatment, the blood cells are then returned to the body. Interleukin has also been combined with infection-fighting lymphocytes (colorless cells produced in lymphoid organs such as the lymph nodes) that have been treated with interleukin-2, creating so-called *lymphokine-activated killer cells* (LAK cells). These cells are then transfused into the patient.

The preliminary results of an even newer way of using IL-2 are very encouraging. One method, called *adoptive immunotherapy,* was initially tested on patients with metastatic melanoma that had spread to the lungs, liver, bone, skin, or tissues under the skin. The treatment involves removing a piece of the tumor and extracting immune-system cells called *tumor-infiltrating lymphocytes* or TILS. The TILS are then grown in IL-2, which boosts their potency. Patients are given a drug to suppress their immune system, and the TILS are then injected into them.

Vaccines

An exciting development in the treatment of patients with advanced melanoma is the use of a vaccine. Its purpose, like that of any vaccine, is to increase a person's immunity against some foreign invader. But in the case of a melanoma vaccine, the specific aim is to boost immunity against the patient's own cancerous cells. This is done with a vaccine developed from substances that are shed by the melanoma cells themselves and then cultured.

A number of scientists have been working on vaccines. Jean-Claude Bystryn, MD, professor of dermatology at the New York University School of Medicine, led a study that produced evidence that a test vaccine can slow the progression of malignant melanoma in some patients. Other scientists have reported similar findings.

It should be made clear that this vaccine is not intended to serve a preventive function for people who have not yet developed melanoma. However, there is hope that a vaccine may someday prove extremely useful in protecting individuals who are at high risk of developing melanoma because of congenital nevi, dysplastic nevi, or a history of sun exposure during childhood and adolescence.

Monoclonal Antibodies

Monoclonal antibodies are preparations of defensive immune-system compounds extracted from human or animal blood cells. These antibodies have been used for several years for diagnostic purposes because of their ability to seek out and lock onto disease organisms. They are used in the diagnosis and (more recently) in the treatment of malignant melanoma.

When monoclonal antibodies are injected into a cancer patient, they seek out and attach themselves to specific proteins, such as those on the surface of cancer cells. The antibodies may then attack the cancer cells, or they may act as carriers, transporting strong chemotherapy drugs or radioactive isotopes directly to the cancer cells without damaging normal cells or causing side effects. Although the treatment is still experimental, skin melanoma has been noted to regress after injection of monoclonal antibodies into lesions.

Other Promising Treatments

Promising treatments used for other cancers are often being tested for malignant melanoma. Some of these may still be experimental (but safe); others may only be available in a limited area of the country. To get the most up-to-date information on what types of clinical trials are available in a community near you, call the NCI at the numbers listed in appendix II.

Spontaneous Regression

An unusual feature of melanoma is that spontaneous regression of the disease occurs in 2.2 out of every 1,000 melanoma patients. Although melanoma accounts for less than 1 percent of all malignancies, it accounts for 11 percent of the documented cases of spontaneous regression in malignancy. These regressions, which are often permanent (thus the patient seems cured) are most frequently on the skin, subcutaneous tissue, lymph nodes, and lungs.

Does this mean that someone with malignant melanoma should take a chance of being among the small percentage of patients who get better without medical intervention? Absolutely not: the odds are not very good, and the stakes are far too high.

Pregnancy After Melanoma

For many years it was believed that melanoma that developed during pregnancy had a more aggressive course than usual melanoma. Patients were often advised not to become pregnant if they had a history of melanoma. More recent studies do not confirm that the relationship between pregnancy and melanoma is as strong as was once believed, however, so most medical oncologists, gynecologists, and dermatologists look at women case by case if pregnancy is being considered. Those with a low-risk melanoma (risk is based on a number of factors considered at the time of diagnosis) may be able to become pregnant safely. Those who are at high risk or who have already experienced a recurrence of the disease are usually advised not to become pregnant. A woman should discuss this with her gynecologist and medical oncologist, as well as with her dermatologist, prior to making a decision to have a baby.

Follow-up

Even when melanoma appears to have been cured by early surgery, patients should continue to be closely monitored by a medical oncologist, who is best able to evaluate any changes that may indicate a recurrence of the disease. Unlike basal cell and squamous cell carcinomas, malignant melanoma is more likely to recur (if it does at all) as a metastatic disease than as another visible skin growth. Melanoma is unpredictable; it can lie dormant for many years, and then suddenly appear elsewhere in the body.

When this occurs, however, it is not a cause for despair. Medical literature reports instances in which individuals have had a recurrence of a malignant melanoma and yet have responded well to treatment. Sometimes a single nodule (small mass or lymph node) develops months or even years after the original primary growth was excised, and removal of the nodule leads to long-term control or cure. Multiple metastases may rule out surgery, but radiation therapy or chemotherapy can still be effective in causing a regression of the disease. Perfusion (discussed earlier) and immunotherapy can also be extremely effective.

Metastatic malignant melanoma is a difficult disease to treat, and unfortunately many people are not cured of it. If you or someone you care about is undergoing treatment for this disease, do not become discouraged. Instead, focus on the knowledge that research continues and that new treatments, as well as new combinations of established treatments, are yielding positive results. Remember, too, that early detection and early treatment can mean total cure.

Emotional Support and Rehabilitation

Skin cancers are generally cured. Malignant melanoma poses a much greater challenge; but here, too, many people who have undergone treatment for it are alive and well.

Still, fear of recurrence is not unusual. It is sometimes difficult to strike a good balance between self-monitoring and regular checkups on the one hand and cancer phobia on the other. Time is often a good emotional healer, and many people are soon able to return to their usual ways of dealing with life. Others may have more difficulty, or they may find that cancer has reminded them of some unresolved issues and concerns in their life. Just as it's never too late to protect yourself from the sun, so it is never too late to try to change feelings, attitudes, behaviors, and relationships. Many people are helped by popular self-help books; others prefer self-help or professionally led groups of people facing similar situations; and some find one-to-one counseling most helpful. Appendixes II and III contain information for getting started in dealing with emotional reactions and stress.

Because treatment for skin cancer often affects the face or another visible part of the anatomy, a person's appearance may be changed. Although the changes may be minimal, they can still be stressful because they alter a person's sense of self.

Such changes can be addressed in two different ways. One way is to try to emphasize your good features and inner self, accepting the external alterations. This may be difficult, but with reassurance from those you care about and sometimes counseling it *can* happen. During my years as a therapist to cancer patients, I've seen many happy, well-adjusted people whose confidence has been restored and whose quality of life is excellent despite disfigurement or scars that would make others miserable.

Another way to cope with cosmetically undesirable results of treatment for skin cancer is to undergo plastic surgery. I never cease to be amazed at the wonderful work plastic surgeons do to correct cosmetic flaws. The dermatologist or surgeon who performed your operation should be able to recommend a well-trained, experienced plastic surgeon whom you can consult. Additional information on how to find a qualified plastic surgeon can be found in appendix II.

Summary

The thought of cancer is frightening to most people, but today's treatments for skin cancer are generally very successful—especially if the problem is detected and treated early, before it has spread.

Dermatologists have various ways of treating and curing basal cell carcinoma and squamous cell carcinoma. Surgery—excisional surgery, electrosurgery, cryosurgery, and laser surgery—plays a significant role in removing malignant lesions. Chemosurgery (better known as *Mohs surgery*) effectively cures people of skin cancers that have grown large or deep or are at high risk of recurring, while sparing as much healthy tissue as possible. Topical chemotherapy, radiation, and immunotherapy may also be effective in treating and curing these cancers.

Melanoma is removed in much the same way as other skin cancers are, but its chances of metastasizing are far greater. If it has already spread at the time of diagnosis, or if it recurs as metastatic disease, prompt treatment is required to achieve the best possible control of it. Standard treatments such as surgery, radiation, chemotherapy, perfusion, and hyperthermia can be used to treat distant sites of tumor. Newer treatments are also being developed, including immunotherapy and vaccines.

Spontaneous regressions have been documented; but although more common in melanoma than in other cancers, they are still infrequent and should not be depended upon, since melanoma is a life-threatening disease.

Women who are free of melanoma after treatment are sometimes advised not to become pregnant; but that once-inflexible rule is now recognized as needing a case-by-case evaluation. Follow-up is essential for everyone who has had skin cancer, since these cancers have a tendency to recur. People who have had cancer often benefit from a setting that provides emotional support; some who have experienced a major change in appearance may wish to consider plastic surgery.

Afterword

An interesting thing happened to me as I began to research and write this book. I became very aware—my husband says "hypervigilant" is more like it—of the effects of the decrease in the ozone layer and of ultraviolet radiation on myself and on everyone else. Not content to wear sunscreen every day, I badgered all those I care about to do the same.

And I became very aware of the environment and how all of us, even in a small way, are part of the problem of pollution. I remembered with guilt all the aerosol cans I used to buy, and I realized that I'm still not as good about recycling as I should be. When my youngest daughter gave birth to a baby in the fall of 1989, I was surprised to learn that she was planning on using cloth diapers; but she explained, "They're nice for Samantha, but they also won't add to pollution like the nonbiodegradable ones they sell in all the stores." How right she is.

And while I worked on this book, I remembered all the wonderful days I spent in the sunshine as a child, and then again as a parent of young children. Would I do it over again? I wouldn't spend summer days indoors, but I would certainly be more careful. I would know how to protect my skin and eyes, and I would stay out of the sun while it is at its strongest.

Am I worried about skin cancer for myself and my family? Not really, because I know enough—and so do they—about how to recognize it early and get prompt treatment. I have some concerns about malignant melanoma because it is difficult to treat if it has spread. But I am encouraged, knowing that none of us plans to "watch a mole grow," but will report any changes or new moles to a dermatologist. And I remember my mother-in-law, who had a melanoma removed from her upper leg in 1964 and lived to see her youngest granddaughter married in 1985, before dying of something else. I am also encouraged by the progress being made in treatment for metastatic melanoma and feel that total control of it isn't far off.

Sometimes when I look in the mirror and see a few more wrinkles than necessary, I ask myself if those glorious days on the beach were worth them. The answer is no. I could have enjoyed the warmth and glow of the sun and still protected myself. But I remember more of my mother's good advice: "Don't look back too often or you'll trip over your feet as you walk forward."

So one day soon I'm going to march myself over to my dermatologist's office and see what's in store for me. Tretinoin perhaps. Collagen injections. Or maybe I'll just stroll over to that nice new cosmetic store that opened in my neighborhood and see what kind of makeup will look best.

And when summer comes around and our eight grandchildren join us in the backyard for fun and sun, there will be sunscreen, hats, and shade to go around.

I now feel completely safe in the sun. You should too.

Mary-Ellen Siegel

Appendixes

Sunscreens Recommended by The Skin Cancer Foundation

The Skin Cancer Foundation grants its seal of recommendation to sunscreen products of SPF 15 or greater that meet the foundation's criteria as "aids in the prevention of sun-induced damage to the skin." Recipients of the seal of recommendation constitute a continually changing list. Each year some products may be deleted, others may be added. Thus we suggest that you send a self-addressed, stamped, envelope requesting the most current listing to: Skin Cancer Foundation, 245 Fifth Avenue, New York, NY 10016.

Reference Guide to Further Information

To Find a Dermatologist, Plastic Surgeon, Opthalmologist or Oncologist

Your personal physician or local hospital should be able to recommend a dermatologist, plastic surgeon, ophthalmologist or medical oncologist. Alternatively, you can call your local medical society and ask for a referral. Most medical societies give three names in response to such requests. The *Directory of Medical Specialists* lists all physicians who are American Board Certified Specialists. A new directory, or a supplement to the existing one, is issued every two years. Many local libraries have the book, or the librarian can suggest where to find it. Dermatologists, ophthalmologists, and plastic surgeons are listed (by community) in the sections entitled "Dermatologists" and "Plastic Surgeons." The credentials or affiliations of any American Board Certified Specialists can be checked by consulting the alphabetical index of the directory.

Most states maintain a medical directory of all state-licensed physicians; this directory is usually available in local libraries. The American Medical Association (AMA) also publishes a directory of physicians in the United States. These books are good sources of information about physicians.

You can also contact the professional organization to which most board-certified dermatologists belong:

American Academy of Dermatology
P.O. Box 1661
Evanston, IL 60204
(312)869-3954

For referral by the AAD to a dermatologist in your area, call 1-(800)-238-2300.

Similarly, you can contact the professional organization to which most physicians certified by the American Board of Plastic Surgery belong:

American Society of Plastic and Reconstructive Surgeons
444 East Algonquin Road
Arlington Heights, IL 60005
(708)228-9900

For referral by the ASPRS to a plastic surgeon in your area, call 1-(800)-635-0635.

To find an ophthalmologist, you can contact the professional organization to which most board-certified ophthalmologists belong:

American Academy of Ophthalmology
P.O. Box 7424
San Francisco, CA 94120-7424
(415)561-8500

For referral to the medical oncologists in your area, contact:

American Society of Clinical Oncologists
435 North Michigan Avenue
Suite 1717
Chicago, IL 60611
(312) 644-0828

Information for Those Concerned About Skin Cancer

Perhaps the best single source of specific materials on skin cancer is the Skin Cancer Foundation:

Skin Cancer Foundation
245 Fifth Avenue
New York, NY 10016
(212)725-5176

This nonprofit organization offers a wide variety of publications on the prevention, diagnosis, and treatment of skin cancer. People are asked to send a stamped, self-addressed envelope for published materials. They also will provide you with their ever-changing current list of sunscreen products that have been approved by the foundation's photobiology committee and thus have received the Skin Cancer Foundation's Seal of Recommendation.

Information for Cancer Patients and Their Families

Cancer Information Service

The National Cancer Institute supports cancer research throughout the country and also conducts their own research. Of special interest and extreme usefulness to cancer patients and their families is the NCI's information and referral service, called the *Cancer Information Service (CIS) of the National Cancer Institutue*. The CIS cn be reached toll-free. In the continental United States, call 1-(800)-4-CANCER. In Hawaii (on Oahu), call 524-1234; call this number collect from neighboring islands).

This nationwide telephone service answers questions from cancer patients and their families. When you call the CIS number you are connected with the regional office serving your area. Counselors there can give you accurate, personalized answers to your cancer-related questions, tell you about various community agencies and services available, and identify the medical library nearest to your home. Upon request, they will give you the name of the closest Comprehensive Cancer Center and tell you where any experimental programs for skin cancer (including melanoma) are being conducted. If you wish, they will guide you in finding a private physician, and in some instances they can give you the names of specific physicians.

Spanish-speaking staff members are available to callers from the following areas (daytime hours only): California, Florida, Georgia, Illinois, northern New Jersey, New York, and Texas.

PDQ

The NCI computerized system known as PDQ (Physician Data Query) gives doctors quick and easy access to the latest treatment information for most types of cancer, to descriptions of clinical trials that are open for patient entry, and to names of organizations and physicians involved in cancer care. Many physicians are able to access PDQ from their office computers, but others use a medical library. Ask your local librarian if a medical library in your community has this service and if it is available to you.

Another NCI resource is the Office of Cancer Communications:

Office of Cancer Communications
National Cancer Institute (NCI)
National Institutes of Health
Building 31, room 10A24
Bethesda, MD 20014

Write to it for a list of available written materials on cancer in general, on skin cancers or melanoma, or on any other specific cancer.

The American Cancer Society (ACS) offers many services as well:

American Cancer Society
National Headquarters
Tower Place
3340 Peachtree Road, N.E.
Atlanta, GA 30026
(404)320-3333

In addition to funding research, the American Cancer Society sponsors several patient support programs. Many local ACS divisions and units can help with transportation to radiation or other medical appointments, and some can help you find and finance care in the home.

Look in your local telephone directory for the nearest American Cancer Society division or unit. Counselors can give you information about locally available services and can provide you with various written materials. If you are unable to find the local division, contact the national office.

If you live in Canada, consult the Canadian Cancer Society:

The Canadian Cancer Society
77 Bloor Street West, suite 1702
Toronto, Ontario, Canada M5S3A1
(416)961-7223

It offers many of the same services as the American Cancer Society and maintains divisions in every province. Check the telephone directory for the division nearest you, or call the national office.

To Find Help in Coping with Diagnosis and Treatment for Skin Cancer

Your physician may be able to refer you to a social worker, psychologist, or psychiatrist who is experienced in helping people cope with disgnosis and treatment of cancer, and with their changing or changed appearance. Self-help groups, sometimes professionally led, may also be available in your community. If your physician can't give you a recommendation, call the social work or psychiatry department of your local hospital or the American or Canadian Cancer Society nearest you for a referral.

Further Reading

AMA. *AMA Family Medical Guide*. New York: Random House, 1987.

AMA Staff. *American Medical Association Encyclopedia of Medicine*. New York: Random House, 1989.

Consumer Reports Books Editors and Richard Waker. *Healthy Skin*. New York: Consumer Reports, 1989.

Jaffe, Hirshel, James Rudin, and Marcia Rudin. *Why Me? Why Anyone?* New York: St. Martin's Press, 1986.

Long, James W. *The Essential Guide to Prescription Drugs, 1990: Everything You Need to Know for Safe Drug Use*. New York: Harper & Row, 1990.

Morgan, Elizabeth, MD. *The Complete Book of Cosmetic Surgery*. New York: Warner, 1988.

Morra, Marion, and Eva Potts. *Choices: Realistic Alternatives in Cancer Treatment*. New York: Avon, 1987.

Nierenberg, Judith, and Florence Janovic. *The Hospital Experience*. New York: Berkley, 1985.

Novick, Nelson. *Skin Care for Teens*. New York: Watts, 1988.

Novick, Nelson. *Super Skin: A Leading Dermatologist's Guide to Head-to-Toe Skin Care*. New York: Crown, 1988.

Pinckney, Cathey, and Edward R. Pinckney, MD. *The Patient's Guide to Medical Tests*. New York: Facts on File, 1986.

Rees, Thomas D., and Sylvia Simmons. *More Than Just a Pretty Face*. Boston: Little, Brown, 1987.

Shulman, Julius M., MD. *Cataracts: The Complete Guide—from Diagnosis to Recovery—for Patients and Families*. Washington, D.C.: American Association for Retired People, 1987.

Siegel, Mary-Ellen. *The Cancer Patient's Handbook*. New York: Walker, 1986.

Subak-Sharpe, Genell, ed. *The Columbia University College of Physicians and Surgeons Complete Home Medical Guide*. New York: Crown, 1989.

Sims, Naomi. *All About Health and Beauty for the Black Woman*. New York: Doubleday, 1986.

U.S. Pharmacopeia. *Drug Information for the Consumer*. 1989 ed. New York: Consumers Reports, 1989.

Winter, Ruth. *Consumer's Dictionary of Cosmetic Ingredients*. Revised ed. New York: Crown, 1989.

Zinn, Walter J., and Herbert Solomon. *The Complete Guide to Eye Care, Eyeglasses and Contact Lenses*. Hollywood, Fla.: Fell, 1987.

Appendix IV
Professional Sources

The assistance of Jaclyn Silverman in compiling these references is gratefully acknowledged.

Azizi, E.; Lusky, A.; Kushelevsky, A. P.; and Schewach-Millet, M. 1988. Skin type, hair color, and freckles are predictors of decreased minimal erythema ultraviolet radiation dose. *J. Amer. Acad. Dermatol.* 19(1): 32–38.

Balin, A. K. 1989. Actinic keratoses. *Skin Cancer Found. J.* 7: 13–81.

Bercovitch, L. 1987. Topical chemotherapy of actinic keratoses of the upper extremity with tretinoin and 5-fluorouracil: A double-blind controlled study. *Br. J. Dermatol.* 116: 549–52.

Bergmanson, J. P.; Pitts, D. G.; and Chu, L. W. 1988. Protection from harmful UV radiation by contact lenses. *J. Amer. Optom. Assoc.* 59(3): 178–82.

Blume, M. R.; Rosenbaum, E. H.; Cohen, R. J.; et al. 1981. Adjuvant immunotherapy of high risk stage I melanoma with transfer factor. *Cancer* 47: 882–88.

Cassiletu, B. R.; Clark, W. H. Jr.; Heiberger, R. M.; March, V.; Tenaglia, A. 1982. Relationship between patients' early recognition of melanoma and depth of invasion. *Cancer.* 49: 198–200.

Council Report. 1989. Harmful effects of ultraviolet radiation. *J. Amer. Med. Assoc.* 262(3): 380–84.

Davies, R. E., and Forbes, P. D. 1988. Retinoids and photocarcinogenesis: A review. *J. Toxicol.* 7: 241–53.

Dilsaver, S. C., and Coffman, J. A. 1988. Seasonal depression. *Amer. Fam. Physician* (October 1988): 173–76.

Dougherty, M. A.; McDermott, R. J.; and Hawkins, M. J. 1987. Those friendly little tanning beds and the public's health. *Amer. J. Public Health* 77(3): 370.

Editorial. 1988. Beauty today and youth tomorrow? *J. Amer. Med. Assoc.* 260: 688–89.

Editorial. 1988. Sunscreens. *Med. Letter* 30(768): 61–63.

Editorial. 1988. Tretinoin for aging skin. *Med. Letter* 30(770): 69–70.

Editorial. 1989. The UV problem: Have the rules changed? *J. Amer. Optom. Assoc.* 60(6): 420–24.

Elwood, J. M.; Cooke, K. R.; Coombs, B. D.; et al. 1988. A strategy for the control of malignant melanoma in New Zealand. *N.Z. Med. J.* 101: 602–4.

Engel, A., and Johnson, M-L. 1988. Health effects of sunlight exposure in the United States: Results from the first national health and nutrition examination survey, 1971–1974. *Arch. Dermatol.* 124: 72–79.

FDA Consumer Report. 1988. FTC puts clouds over fake tanning claims. Federal Trade Commission, March 1988, p. 5.

FDA Consumer Report. 1989. Burns, eye injuries from tanning devices. Federal Trade Commission, October 1989, p. 3.

Fears, T. R., and Scotto, J. 1986. Estimated increase in skin cancer morbidity due to increase in ultraviolet radiation exposure. *Cancer Invest.* 1: 119–26.

Fleming, I. D.; Barnawell, J. R.; Burlison, P. E.; and Rankin, J. S. 1975. Skin cancer in black patients. *Cancer* 35: 600–5.

Freeman, N. R.; Fairbrother, G. E.; and Rose, R. J. 1982. Survey of skin cancer incidence in the Hamilton area. *N.Z. Med. J.* 95: 529–33.

Friedman, H. S., and Keesling, B. 1989. Experimental evaluation of interventions to prevent skin cancer. Paper presented at 10th annual meeting of the Society of Behavioral Medicine, San Francisco, CA, April 1989.

Gange, R. W. 1987. Acute effects of ultraviolet radiation in the skin. In T. B. Fitzpatrick, A. Z. Eisen, K. Wolff, et al., eds., *Dermatology in General Medicine.* 3d ed. New York: McGraw-Hill, pp. 1451–57.

Gilchrest, B. A. 1988. At last! A medical treatment for skin aging. *J. Amer. Med. Assoc.* 259(4): 569–70.

Glass, A. G., and Hoover, R. N. 1989. The emerging epidemic of melanoma and squamous cell skin cancer. *J. Amer. Med. Assoc.* 262(15): 1097–100.

Goette, D. K. 1981. Topical chemotherapy with 5-fluorouracil: A review. *J. Amer. Acad. Dermatol.* 4: 633–49.

Goldsmith, M. F. 1987. Medical news & perspectives: Paler is better, say skin cancer fighters. *J. Amer. Med. Assoc.* 257(7): 893–94.

———. 1987. Medical news & perspectives: Unusual moles play

leading role in new strategies for predicting and preventing malignant melanoma. *J. Amer. Med. Assoc.* 257(7): 894–95.

Green, A. 1982. Incidence and reporting of cutaneous melanoma in Queensland. *Aust. J. Derm.* 23: 105–9.

Green, M. H.; Clark, W. H., Jr.; Tucker, M. A.; et al. 1985. High risk of malignant melanoma in melanoma-prone families with dysplastic nevi. *Ann. Intern. Med.* 102: 458–65.

Halpern, A. 1989. Malignant melanoma: Early detection improves prognosis. *Skin Cancer Found. J.* 7: 33–71.

Hanke, W. C.; Zollinger, T. W.; O'Brian, J. J.; and Bianco, L. 1985. Skin cancer in professional and amateur female golfers. *Physician and Sportsmedicine* 13(8): 51–68.

Hill, D.; Rassaby, J.; and Gardner, G. 1984. Determinants of intentions to take precautions against skin cancer. *Community Health Studies* 8: 33–44.

Holly, E. A.; Kelly, J. W.; Shpall, S. N.; and Chiu, S-H. 1987. Number of melanocytic nevi as a major risk factor for malignant melanoma. *J. Amer. Acad. Dermatol.* 17: 459–68.

Holman, C. D.; Armstrong, B. K.; and Heenan, P. J. 1986. Relationship of cutaneous malignant melanoma to individual sun exposure habits. *J. Nat. Cancer Inst.* 76: 403–14.

Horgan, J. 1988. Skin saver: Researchers seek a vaccine to treat and prevent melanoma. *Scientific Amer.* 2: 40.

Hurwitz, S. 1988. The sun and sunscreen protection: Recommendations for children. *J. Dermatol. Surg. Oncol.* 14(6): 657–60.

Jacobsen, F. M.; Wehr, T. A.; Sack, D. A.; James, S. P.; and Rosenthal, N. E. 1987. Seasonal affective disorder: A review of the syndrome and its public health implications. *Amer. J. Public Health* 77(1): 57–60.

Jaworsky, C.; Ratz, J. L.; and Dijkstra, J. W. E. 1987. Efficacy of tan accelerators. *J. Amer. Acad. Dermatol.* 16(4): 769–71.

Keesling, B., and Friedman, H. S. 1987. Psychosocial factors in sunbathing and sunscreen use. *Health Psychol.* 6: 477–93.

Kligman, A. M. 1969. Early destructive effects of sunlight on human skin. *J. Amer. Med. Assoc.* 210: 2377–80.

Kligman, A. M.; Grove, G. L.; Hirose, H.; and Leyden, J. J. 1986.

Topical tretinoin for photoaged skin. *J. Amer. Acad. Dermatol.* 15: 836–59.

Kligman, A. M., and Lavker, R. M. 1988. Cutaneous aging: The differences between intrinsic aging and photoaging. *J. Cutaneous Aging Cosmet. Dermatol.* 1: 1.

Kligman, L. H. 1989. Photoaging manifestations, prevention, and treatment. *Clin. Geriat. Med.* 5: 235–51.

Kligman, L. H.; Atkin, F. J.; and Kligman, A. M. 1983. Sunscreens promote repair of ultraviolet-induced dermal damage. *J. Invest. Dermatol.* 81: 98–102.

Kligman, L. H., and Kligman, A. M. 1986. The nature of photoaging: Its prevention and repair. *Photodermatology* 3(4) 215–27.

Kopf, A. W.; Rivers, J. K.; Slue, W.; Rigel, D. S.; and Friedman, R. J. 1988. Photographs are useful for detection of malignant melanomas in patients who have dysplastic nevi. *J. Amer. Acad. Dermatol.* 19(6): 1132–34.

Kraemer, K. H.; Tucker, M.; Tarone, R.; Elder, D. E.; and Clark, W. H., Jr. 1986. Risk of cutaneous melanoma in dysplastic nevus syndrome types A and B. *N. Eng. J. Med.* 315: 1615.

Kripke, M. L. 1984. Immunological unresponsiveness induced by ultraviolet radiation. *Immunol. Rev.* 80: 878–902.

———. 1986. Immunology and photocarcinogenesis. *J. Amer. Acad. Dermatol.* 14:149–55.

Kuflik, E. G.; Lubritz, R. R.; and Torre, D. 1984. Cryosurgery. *Dermatol. Clin.* 2: 319–32.

Leffell, D. J. 1989. From chicks to skin: Vitamin A and cancer. *Skin Cancer Found. J.* 7: 13–81.

Lew, R. A.; Sober, A. J.; Cook, N.; et al. 1983. Sunburn, sun exposure, and melanoma skin cancer. *J. Dermatol. Surg. Oncol.* 9: 981–86.

Lippman, S. M.; Kessler, J. F.; and Meyskens, F. L. 1987. Retinoids as preventive and therapeutic anticancer agents. Part I. *Cancer Treat. Rep.* 71: 391–405.

———. 1987. Retinoids as preventive and therapeutic anticancer agents. Part II. *Cancer Treat. Rep.* 71: 493–515.

Lippman, S. M., and Meyskens, F. L. 1987. Treatment of advanced squamous cell carcinoma of the skin with isotretinoin. *Ann. Intern. Med.* 107: 499–501.

Longstreth, J. D. 1987. Ultraviolet radiation and melanoma with a special focus on assessing the risks of stratospheric ozone depletion. Washington, DC: U.S. Government Printing Office.

Lowe, N. J.; Dromgoole, S. H.; Sefton, J.; et al. 1987. Indoor and outdoor efficacy testing of a broad-spectrum sunscreen against ultraviolet A radiation in psoralen-sensitized subjects. *J. Amer. Acad. Dermatol.* 17(2): 224–30.

Marks, R.; Kennie, G.; and Selwood, T. S. 1988. Malignant transformation of solar keratoses to squamous cell carcinoma. *Lancet* 1: 795–97.

Marks, R. 1989. Skin cancer in Australia. *Skin Cancer Found. J.* 7: 9–57.

Mastrangelo, M. J.; Baker, A. R.; and Katx, H. R. 1985. Cutaneous melanoma. In V. T. DeVita, Jr., S. Hellman, S. A. Rosenberg, eds. *Cancer, Principles and Practice of Oncology.* 2d ed. Philadelphia: Lippincott, pp. 1371–1422.

Matsuoka, L. Y.; Ide, L.; Wortsman, J.; et al. 1987. Sunscreens suppress cutaneous vitamin D_3 synthesis. *J. Clin. Endocrinol. Metab.* 64: 1165–68.

Meyskens, F. L., Jr.; Edwards, L.; and Levine, N. S. 1986. Role of topical tretinoin in melanoma and dysplastic nevi. *J. Amer. Acad. Dermatol.* 15: 822–25.

Mikhail, G. R., and Gorsulowsky, D. C. 1986. Spontaneous regression of metastatic malignant melanoma. *J. Dermatol. Surg. Oncol.* 12: 497–500.

Mohs. F. E. 1986. Micrographic surgery for the microscopically controlled excision of eyelid cancers. *Arch. Ophthalmol.* 104: 901–9.

Mora, R. G., and Burris, R. 1981. Cancer of the skin in blacks: A reivew of 128 patients with basal-cell carcinoma. *Cancer* 47: 1436–38.

Mora, R. G., and Perniciaro, C. 1981. Cancer of the skin in blacks: I. A review of 163 black patients with cutaneous squamous cell carcinoma. *J. Amer. Acad. Dermatol.* 5: 535–43.

Mora, R. G.; Perniciaro, C.; and Lee, B. 1984. Cancer of the skin in blacks: III. A review of nineteen black patients with Bowen's disease. *J. Amer. Acad. Dermatol.* 11: 557–62.

NIH Consensus Development Conference. 1989. Sunlight, untraviolet radiation, and the skin. Warren Grant Magnuson Clinical Center, May 8–10, 1989.

Olson, C. M. 1989. Increased outdoor recreation, diminished ozone layer pose ultraviolet radiation threat to eye. *J. Amer. Med. Assoc.* 261(8): 1102–3.

Pathak, M. A., and Robins, P. 1989. A response to concerns about sunscreens. *Skin Cancer Found. J.* 7: 54–55.

Peck, G. L. 1986. Topical tretinoin in actinic keratosis and basal cell carcinoma. *J. Amer. Acad. Dermatol.* 5: 829–35.

Pitts, D. G., and Bergmanson, J. P. G. 1989. The UV problem: Have the rules changed? *J. Amer. Optom. Assoc.* 60(6): 420–24.

Rampen, F. H. J.; van der Meeren, H. L. M.; and Boezeman, J. B. M. 1986. Frequency of moles as a key to melanoma incidence? *J. Amer. Acad. Dermatol.* 15(6): 1200–3.

Rampen, F. H. J.; Fleuren, B. A. M.; de Boo, T. M.; Lemmens, W. A. J. G. 1988. Unreliability of self-reported burning tendency and tanning ability. *Arch. Dermatol.* 124: 885–88.

Rapp, F. B.; Dorsey, S. B.; and Guin, J. D. 1987. The tanning salon: An area survey of equipment, procedures and practices. *J. Amer. Acad. Dermatol.* 18: 1030–38.

Rege, V.; Leone, L.; Soderberg, C.; et al. 1987. Hyperthermic perfusion for stage I malignant melanoma of the extremity. *Proc. Amer. Soc. Clin. Oncol.* 6: 211.

Renneker, M. 1987. Medical aspects of surfing. *Physician and Sportsmedicine* 15(12): 96–105.

Rhodes, A. R., and Fitzpatrick, T. B. 1983. Melanoma precursors: Risk factors and opportunities for prevention of cutaneous melanomas. *J. Dermatol. Surg. Oncol.* 9: 672–73.

Rhodes, A. R.; Weinstock, M. A.; Fitzpatrick, T. B.; et al. 1987. Risk factors for cutaneous melanoma: A practical method of recognizing predisposed individuals. *J. Amer. Med. Assoc.* 258: 3146–54.

Rigel, D. S.; Friedman, R. J.; Kopf, A. W.; et al. 1986. Importance of complete cutaneous examination for the detection of malignant melanoma. *J. Amer. Acad. Dermatol.* 14: 857–60.

Rigel, D. S.; Rivers, J. K.; Friedman, R. J.; and Kopf, A. W. 1988.

Risk gradient for malignant melanoma in individuals with dysplastic nevi. *Lancet* 1: 352–53.

Rigel, D. S.; Rivers, J. K.; Kopf, A. W.; et al. 1989. Dysplastic nevi: Markers for increased risk for melanoma. *Cancer* 63: 386–89.

Robins, P. 1989. The most common cancer: Basal cell carcinoma. *Skin Cancer Found. J.* 7: 29–69.

Robinson, J. K. 1987. Risk of developing another basal cell carcinoma: A 5-Year prospective study. *Cancer* 60: 118–20.

Rosenberg, S.; Lotze, M. T.; Muul, L. M.; et al. 1987. A progress report on the treatment of 157 patients with advanced cancer using lymphokine-activated killer cells and interleukin-2 or high-dose interleukin-2 alone. *N. Eng. J. Med.* 316: 889–97.

Rosenthal, F. S.; Phoon, C.; Bakalian, A. E.; and Taylor, H. R. 1988. The ocular dose of ultraviolet radiation to outdoor workers. *Invest. Ophthal. & Vis. Science* 29(4): 649–56.

Sams, W. M. 1986. Sun-induced aging. *Dermatol. Clinics* 4(3): 509–16.

———. 1989. Sun-induced aging: Clinical and laboratory observations in humans. *Clin. Geriat. Med.* 5: 223–33.

Schwartz, R. A. 1988. *Skin Cancer: Recognition and Management.* New York: Springer-Verlag.

Silverberg, E. 1989. Cancer statistics, 1989. *CA* 39: 3–20.

Stern, R. S., and Docken, W. 1986. An exacerbation of SLE after visiting a tanning salon. *J. Amer. Med. Assoc.* 256: 3120.

Stern, R. S.; Lange, R.; et al. 1988. Non-melanoma skin cancer occurring in patients treated with PUVA five to ten years after first treatment. *J. Invest. Dermatol.* 91: 120–24.

Stern. R. S.; Weinstein, M. C.; and Baker, S. G. 1986. Risk reduction for nonmelanoma skin cancer with childhood sunscreen use. *Arch. Dermatol.* 122: 537–45.

Stiehm, E. R.; Kronenberg, L. H.; Rosenblatt, H. M.; et al. 1982. Interferon: Immunobiology and clinical significance. *Ann. Intern. Med.* 96: 80–93.

Stolarski, R. S. 1988. The Antarctic ozone hole. *Scientific Amer.* 258: 30–36.

Stoll, H. L., Jr., and Schwartz, R. A. 1987. Squamous cell carcinoma.

In T. B. Fitzpatrick, A. Z. Eisen, K. Wolff, et al., eds., *Dermatology in General Medicine*. 3d ed. New York: McGraw-Hill, pp. 746–58.

Taylor, H. K.; West, S. K.; Rosenthal, F. S.; et al. 1988. Effect of ultraviolet radiation on cataract formation. *N. Eng. J. Med.* 319: 1429–33.

Torre, D. 1986. Cryosurgery of basal cell carcinoma. *J. Amer. Acad. Dermatol.* 15: 917–29.

Tucker, M. A.; Shields, J. A.; Hartge, P.; Augsburger, J.; Hoover, R. N.; Fraumeni, J. F. 1985. Sunlight Exposure as Risk Factor For Intraocular Malignant Melanoma. *J. Amer. Med. Assoc.* 343(13): 789–792.

Ullrich, S. E., and Kripke, M. L. 1989. Effects of ultraviolet radiation on the immune system. *Skin Cancer Found. J.* 7: 37–97.

Vance, C. J. 1989. Interferon treatment of skin cancers. *Skin Cancer Found. J.* 7: 19–67.

Walters, B. L., and Kelley, T. M. 1987. Commercial tanning facilities: A new source of eye injury. *Amer. J. Emerg. Med.* 5(5): 386–89.

Webb, A. R., and Holick, M. F. 1988. The role of sunlight in the cutaneous production of vitamin D_3. *Ann. Rev. Nutr.* 8: 376–99.

Weinstock, M. A. 1989. The epidemic of squamous cell carcinoma. *J. Amer. Med. Assoc.* 262(15): 2138–39.

Weinstock, M. A.; Colditz, G. A.; Willett, W. C.; et al. 1989. Nonfamilial cutaneous melanoma incidence in women associated with sun exposure before 20 years of age. *Pediatrics* 84: 199–204.

Weiss, J. S.; Ellis, C. N.; Headington, J. T.; Tincoff, T.; Hamilton, M. S.; Voorhees, J. 1988. Topical tretinoin improves photodamaged skin: A double-blind vehicle-controlled study. *J. Amer. Med. Assoc.* 259: 527–32.

Weiss, J. S.; Ellis, C. N.; Headington, J. T.; et al. 1988. Topical tretinoin in the treatment of aging skin. *J. Amer. Acad. Dermatol.* 19(1): 169–75.

Wiley, H. E. 1989. Don't take the small fry lightly. *Skin Cancer Found. J.* 7: 7–65.

Glossary

ACTINIC KERATOSIS. A precancerous condition that may begin as smooth, flat, or slightly raised pink spots that eventually become irregular, scaly, and wartlike and turn red or brownish in color. Usually occur in sun-exposed areas. Also called solar or senile keratoses.

ACUTE. Rapidly developing, quick, sudden.

ALBINISM. Condition of being born with partial or total lack of melanin pigment. Albinos are prone to severe sunburn, skin inflammations, rashes, and skin cancer, following *any* exposure to ultraviolet radiation. Total albinos have pale skin, white hair, and pink eyes that are abnormally sensitive to light. Albinos are represented in all racial and ethnic groups.

ANALGESIC. A drug that can relieve pain without anesthesia or loss of consciousness. Mild analgesics include aspirin and similar products, many of which do not require a prescription.

ANESTHETIC. A substance that causes loss of sensation in all or part of the body. General anesthetic causes lack of consciousness and sensation. Local anesthetic causes only lack of sensation.

ANGIOGRAM. A diagnostic radiology test during which dye is introduced into the body so that the vessel structures and arteries leading to various organs are made visible. Also called an *arteriogram*.

ANSI SUNGLASS STANDARD. A voluntary labeling program carried out by the Sunglass Association of America, an industry group that worked together with the FDA to provide consumers with uniform, sound, and useful labeling for nonprescription sunglasses. The ANSI standard, placed on a label attached to sunglasses, describes how much ultraviolet radiation is blocked out.

ANTERIOR. Front.

ANTIBODY. Part of the body's own defense formed in response to an antigen. Antibodies help defend the body against infection or toxic substances.

ANTIGEN. A substance, foreign to the body's system, that induces resistance to infection or toxic substance.

AUTOIMMUNITY. A condition in which the body's immune system produces antibodies to fight its own tissues and substances.

BACTERIA. A broad class of one-celled microorganisms, some of which must live and feed off other living things. Many (but not all) bacteria are capable of causing disease.

BASAL CELL CARCINOMA (BCC). The most common type of skin cancer. It grows slowly, seldom spreads beneath the skin, and is easily cured—especially if treated promptly.

BASAL CELLS. Small round cells found in the lowest (innermost) part of the epidermis.

B CELLS. Manufactured in the bone marrow, these cells produce antibodies that help defend the body against infection or toxic substances.

BENIGN. Characteristic of a mild illness or a nonmalignant growth. A benign (or nonmalignant) tumor is one that does not invade and destroy neighboring normal tissue.

BIOPSY. A procedure whereby tissue is removed from living patients for further study, to aid the physician in making a medical diagnosis.

BLOOD CELLS. Cells that, together with plasma, make up blood. Manufactured in bone marrow, they include red blood cells, white blood cells, and platelets.

BLOOD COUNT. Calculation of the number of red cells, white cells, and platelets in a given sample of blood. Taking a blood count aids in the diagnosis of a disease or deficiency.

BLOODSTREAM. Flowing blood in the circulatory system.

BLOOD TRANSFUSION. Introduction of whole blood or some specific component of blood (red blood cells, white blood cells, plasma, or platelets) into the circulation to replace lost blood or to correct deficiencies.

BOARD-CERTIFIED SPECIALIST. A physician who has received formal training in a medical or surgical specialty and then passed the relevant examination.

BODY IMAGING. Any examination technique that gives a picture of the body's interior. Examples include X rays, nuclear scans, CT scans, ultrasound, and MRI.

BONE SCAN. A picture of the bones obtained by a process that involves first injecting the patient with a radioactive chemical that travels to the areas around the bone, highlighting any bone injury, repair, or destruction. This is an extremely sensitive test, useful in diagnosing cancer that has spread to the bones.

BOWEN'S DISEASE. Alternately described as a precancerous condition or as a rare form of cancer. It appears as a scaling, reddish pink, raised growth, usually on unexposed areas of the skin.

CANCER. The uncontrolled growth of abnormal cells. Also called *malignant neoplasm* or *malignancy*.

CARCINOMA. Cancers that begin in tissues that cover or line the body or internal organs.

CARCINOMA IN SITU. A premalignant growth of cancer that is still confined to the tissue where it originated.

CATARACT. A change in the structure of the lens in the eye that leads to any loss of transparency for any reason.

CHEMICAL PEEL. A controlled burning of the skin in which a caustic chemical is applied to remove the primary (top) layer and part of the secondary layer of skin. The old skin remains in place until a new skin has formed underneath it.

CHEMOSURGERY. *See* MOHS SURGERY.

CHEMOTHERAPY. Treatment of illness by drugs or medication that can reach all parts of the body. The term is most often used to describe the treatment of cancer by drugs that can interfere with cancer cell growth and destroy cancer cells.

CHOROID. A delicate membrane layer of the eye lying between the sclera and the retina. It is continuous with the iris and the ciliary body in front of it.

CILIARY BODY. A vascular and muscular structure lying between the choroid layer and the iris.

CLINICAL TRIAL. A study conducted to evaluate a new treatment.

COLLAGEN. A natural protein constituent of connective tissue in humans and other vertebrates. Injectable collagen is a natural animal protein made from the skin of cattle and injected into the skin to eliminate wrinkles or facial depressions.

COMPLETE BLOOD COUNT (CBC). *See* BLOOD COUNT.

CONGENITAL NEVUS. *See* NEVUS.

CONJUCTIVA. Membrane that covers the exposed front portion of the sclera and continues to form the lining of the inside of the eyelid.

CONTRAST MEDIUM. A dye injected or gradually flowed into a vein to highlight internal structures for visualization through X rays or other body-imaging techniques.

CORNEA. Membrane that covers and protects the iris. Sensitive, but tough, it is an extension of the sclera at the front of the eye.

CRYOSURGERY. Surgery that makes use of an extremely low-temperature probe.

CT SCAN. *See* TOMOGRAPHY.

CURETTAGE. Removal of one or more growths with a curette.

CURETTE. A spoon-shaped instrument with a sharp edge, used to remove growths from the skin.

DERMABRASION. A controlled burning of the skin by chemicals, as a result of which the top layer of skin is removed.

DERMATOLOGIST. A physician who specializes in diagnosing and treating skin problems.

DERMIS. The lower layer of the skin, beneath the epidermis.

DIAGNOSIS. The process of determining the nature of a disease so that it can be properly treated.

DINITROCHLOROBENZENE (DNCB). A chemical applied to skin in cream form to eliminate some skin cancers.

DISCOID LUPUS ERYTHEMATOSUS (DLE). Chronic, recurrent disease, primarily of the skin, characterized by a red, scaly, butterfly-like pattern covering the cheeks and the bridge of the nose. It can also occur on other parts of the body. Individuals with DLE tend to be photosensitive. *See also* SYSTEMIC LUPUS ERYTHEMATOSUS.

DYSPLASTIC NEVUS. *See* NEVUS.

-ECTOMY. Suffix meaning "surgical removal" (of the body part specified in the preceding part of word, as in *appendectomy*).

ECZEMA. Skin rash, often very itchy, that may be improved or worsened by exposure to the sun.

ELECTRODESSICATION. Form of electrosurgery in which tissue is destroyed by being burned with an electric spark. Also called *fulguration*.

ELECTROSURGERY. Destruction of tissue through the use of high-frequency electric current.

ENUCLEATION. Surgical removal of the entire eyeball.

EPIDERMIS. The surface layer of the skin.

EXCISION. Surgical removal of tissue or a body part.

FDA (FOOD AND DRUG ADMINISTRATION). Government regulatory agency.

FIBRIL. Synthetic substance that can be injected into wrinkles and depressions to smooth them out.

FLUOROURACIL. An anticancer drug often used on the skin. Also known as *5-fluorouracil* and *5-FU*.

FOLLICLES. Shafts through which hair grows.

FTC (FEDERAL TRADE COMMISSION). Government regulatory agency.

FULGURATION. *See* ELECTRODESSICATION.

GALLIUM SCAN. A nuclear scan that can enable the viewer to identify rapidly dividing cells and to detect lymph node involvement.

GLAND. An organ that selectively removes material from the bloodstream and converts it into a new substance, which either may be recirculated through the bloodstream for a specific function or may be excreted.

HEATSTROKE. A condition in which the body's temperature has risen to a dangerously high level resulting in hot, dry skin, no sweating, along with a high body temperature, weakness, dizziness, rapid breathing, nausea, and sometimes mental confusion or unconsciousness. It is imperative to cool the person quickly.

HORMONE. A chemical substance formed in one part of the body (usually in an endocrine gland) that is carried in the blood to other body parts. When hormones are secreted into body fluids, they have a specific effect on other organs.

HYPERPIGMENTATION. Greater (and thus darker) pigmentation than usual on a given body. Black skin often responds to trauma with hyperpigmentation, but the phenomenon occurs in all racial and ethnic groups.

HYPERTHERMIA. Treatment in which heat is applied to the entire body, to a part of it, or to a tumor alone. *See also* PERFUSION.

HYPERTROPHIC SCARS. A condition in which excessive tissue, in the form of scars, rises about the skin. Often referred to as "proud flesh."

HYPOPIGMENTATION. Loss of pigmentation, with consequent lightening of skin. Black skin often responds to trauma with hypopigmentation, but the phenomenon occurs in all racial and ethnic groups.

IMMUNE SYSTEM. The group of cells and organs evolved to defend the body from foreign substances that might cause infection or disease.

IMMUNOTHERAPY. Treatment directed at producing immunity or resistance to a disease or condition.

INTERFERON. A substance released naturally by animals and humans in response to invading viruses. Now produced synthetically as well as naturally, it can in some instances recognize, suppress, and/or destroy cancer cells and can trigger further defensive responses by the immune system.

INTERLEUKIN. A substance naturally formed by some white blood cells called T Cells. It can also be synthesized in the laboratory. Also called interleukin-2 or IL2.

INTRAOCULAR LENS (IOL). A small, plastic lens that is surgically placed within the eye at the time of cataract removal to restore the focusing power that had been provided by the eye's natural lens before the cataract developed.

INTRAOCULAR MELANOMA. Melanoma of the eye. It usually begins in the pigment-forming cells of the iris, the ciliary body, or the choroid.

ISOLATED PERFUSION. Chemotherapy treatment in which the affected area is isolated by means of a tourniquet, and then drugs are administered directly into it. This procedure may be used to treat malignant malanoma. Also called *hyperthermia profusion*.

KELOID. Large, permanent, and sometimes deforming scars that may develop following surgery or any injury to the skin.

KERATIN. A fibrous protein that is the end product of maturing cells in the stratum corneum.

KERATITIS. Inflammation of the cornea.

KERATOCONJUNCTIVITIS. Combined inflammation of the cornea and conjunctiva, amounting to a severe case of sunburn of the eyes. Often called *snow blindness.*

LAK CELLS. (Lymphokine-activated killer cells) Produced by combining interleukin with infection-fighting lymphocytes that have been treated with interleukin-2, then transfused into a patient.

LANGERHANS CELLS. Part of the immune system that fight off foreign substances such as bacteria, viruses, and allergens.

LASER. Acronym for *Light Amplification by Stimulated Emission of Radiation.* A laser beam is an extremely concentrated source of light; it emits so much heat that it can destroy anything in its path.

LENS. Flexible structure of the eye that allows light to pass through it and focuses the light by altering its shape. The lens refracts or bends light and sends the images to the retina.

LESION. A mass of cells that may be solid, semisolid (cystic), inflammatory, benign, or malignant. The term also applies to a lump or abscess.

LIVER SPOTS. *See* SOLAR LENTIGINES.

LOCALIZED. Remaining at the site of origin.

LUPUS. *See* DISCOID LUPUS ERYTHEMATOSUS AND SYSTEMIC LUPUS ERYTHEMATOSUS

LYMPH. A clear, watery, sometimes faintly yellowish liquid containing lymphocytes, white blood cells, and some red blood cells. It travels through the lymph system to remove bacteria from tissues, transport fat from intestines, and supply lymphocytes to blood.

LYMPHANGIOGRAM. A diagnostic test used to inspect lymph glands.

LYMPHATIC SYSTEM. The interconnected circulatory system of spaces and vessels that carry lymph throughout the body.

LYMPH NODES. Structures throughout the body that contain lymph. They also act as a defense system, triggering an immune response to cancer as well as to bacteria and viruses. They are often the first area of the body to which cancer spreads.

LYMPHOCYTES. Colorless cells produced in lymphoid organs such as the lymph nodes, spleen, and thymus. Their purpose is to fight infection.

MACULA. The high-resolution or fine-tuning part of the eye's retina, needed for close work.

MACULAR DEGENERATION. A progressive condition in which the macula gets thinner and its cells degenerate. In some instances, leakage occurs from small blood vessels that grow in the macular region.

MAGNETIC RESONANT IMAGING (MRI). A diagnostic technique that produces a body-section image and can detect dead or degenerating cells, blockage of blood flow, and cancer.

MALIGNANT. Cancerous.

MALIGNANT TUMOR. A growth of cancer cells.

MELANIN. Pigment of the skin that accounts for variations in skin color.

MELANOCYTES. Cells that produce and contain melanin. They are found in the basal layer of the skin.

MELANOMA. Cancer that originates from melanocytes. Malignant melanoma often begins as a dark mole. Unlike the more common skin cancers, malignant melanoma tends to spread to internal organs if left unchecked.

METASTASIS. The shifting or spread of an original cancerous tumor to another part of the body. The transplantation usually occurs through the bloodstream or the lymph system.

METASTATIC LESION. A small patch of malignant tissue (or tumor) that has spread from the original site of cancer, however remote.

MICROSCOPIC. Too small to be visible to the naked eye, but large enough to be visible under a microscope.

MODALITY. Method of treatment.

MOHS SURGERY. A form of surgery for skin cancer in which cancerous skin and some surrounding area is removed and then microscopically examined. If cancerous cells are present, the procedure is repeated, until microscopical examination indicates that no cancer cells remain.

MOLE. *See* NEVI.

MONITOR. To watch closely.

MONOCLONAL ANTIBODIES. Preparations of defensive immune-system compounds extracted from human or animal blood cells. Used for several years for diagnostic purposes, they are now used for treatment purposes as well.

MRI. *See* MAGNETIC RESONANCE IMAGING.

NATURAL KILLER (NK) CELLS. Stimulated by viral infections, the natural resistance they confer differ from the immunity acquired through previous exposure and is not caused by B or T cells.

NEOPLASM. A tumor or abnormal growth or swelling of tissue. It may be benign or malignant, although the term usually refers to the latter.

NEVUS. A mole, which is a common small blemish or growth on the skin, sometimes referred to as a beauty mark, and which appears in the first few decades of life in most people. Most nevi are normal and are acquired during the first thirty years of life. *Congenital nevus* refers to a mole that is present at birth or that develops by the time a baby is six months old; such moles tend to run in families. *Dysplastic nevi* refers to abnormal moles that may develop anytime in life; people who have them have a susceptibility to developing malignant melanoma. The tendency to develop such nevi may not be inherited.

NONMELANOMA SKIN CANCER. Skin cancer that does not involve melanocytes. Basal cell carcinoma and squamous cell carcinoma are nonmelanoma skin cancers.

NODULE. A small mass of tissue or a tumor, usually malignant.

NUCLEAR MEDICINE. A specialty based on training in nuclear imaging tests. Physicians who specialize in nuclear medicine are also trained in internal medicine, pathology, and radiology.

NUCLEAR SCAN. A diagnostic test that makes use of a small amount of one or more radioactive trace compounds.

OCCLUSIVE DRESSING. A dressing that prevents air from reaching a wound or lesion and that retains moisture, heat, body fluids, and medication.

-OMA. Suffix meaning "tumor" (as in *melanoma*).

ONCOGENES. Cancer genes, which may be associated with changes in chromosomes that alter normal genes into becoming cancerous.

ONCOLOGIST. A physician specifically trained to treat cancer. Medical oncologists usually treat patients with chemotherapy and often are responsible for coordinating the overall treatment of the cancer patient. Surgical oncologists specialize in the surgical treatment of cancer patients. Radiation oncologists specialize in the use of radiotherapy for cancer patients.

ONCOLOGY. The study and treatment of cancer.

OPHTHALMOLOGIST. A medical doctor who is educated, trained, and licensed to provide complete medical eye care, including surgery.

ORALLY. By mouth.

ORGAN. A structural collection of tissues and cells that together perform one or more particular functions. Examples include the liver, the spleen, the digestive organs, and the reproductive organs.

OZONE LAYER. An outer atmospheric layer that contains an unusually high concentration of ozone (O_3) a form of molecular oxygen. Over 99 percent of the earth's atmosphere lies beneath this layer. Because the ozone layer absorbs most ultraviolet radiation from the sun that would otherwise strike the earth, any decrease in it poses a threat to life.

PALLIATIVE TREATMENT. Treatment that is aimed not at a cure but at making a patient feel better by relieving symptoms, pain, or discomfort caused by a disease.

PARA-AMINOBENZOIC ACID (PABA). A chemical used in some sunscreening products. Some people are allergic to it.

PATHOLOGIST. A physician who studies cells and tissues removed from the body, and then makes a diagnosis based on these results.

PATHOLOGY. A branch of medicine that deals with the results of disease, particularly as seen in cell, organ, and tissue changes.

PERFUSION. A procedure in which a high dose of chemotherapy is administered into an extremity. *See also Isolated perfusion* and *Regional perfusion.*

PHACOEMULSIFICATION. A method of cataract removal that utilizes ultrasound technology and requires only a very small incision of the eye. The cataract is broken up into small pieces while still inside the eye; then it is sucked out through a tiny hole by a vibrating titanium needle.

PHOTOAGING. Obvious and microscopic skin changes that result from exposure to ultraviolet radiation.

PHOTOALLERGY. An adverse reaction by the body's immune system to some chemical, following exposure to ultraviolet radiation. Some ingredients in cosmetics and sunscreens are photoallergens for a number of people

PHOTOSENSITIVITY. An adverse response (rash, redness, and/or swelling) to sunlight (UVR) resulting from an interaction between the sun (or ultraviolet radiation) and certain medications. Some people suffer from photosensitivity without having taken any medication.

PLASTIC SURGEON. A physician who is trained and specializes in performing surgery to minimize scarring and disfigurement that may result from any number of causes, including skin cancer.

POLYCARBONATE. An impact-resistant, UVR-blocking plastic that can be used for prescription and nonprescription eyewear.

POLYMORPHOUS LIGHT ERUPTION (PMLE). A disorder that causes an abnormal response to ultraviolet radiation.

PORPHYRIA. Any of a group of inherited disorders in which the body abnormally makes certain parts of the hemoglobin molecule (located in the red blood cells). The resulting substances act as photosensitizers and can cause erosions, scars, and severe hyperpigmentation.

POSTERIOR. Back or rear.

PRIMARY TUMOR. Original tumor. Even if a tumor spreads to form a secondary or metastatic tumor, it continues to be called by the name of the primary or original tumor.

PROGNOSIS. The doctor's forecast of the probable outcome of a disease.

PROPHYLAXIS. Prevention of or protection against a disease or its complications.

PROTOCOL. Written, predetermined treatment plan that specifies the drugs or treatments a patient will receive, their doses, and their frequency. The term also refers to a scientific study designed to determine the most effective treatment for a specific type of cancer or disease.

PSORALEN. A light-sensitizing medication administered prior to exposure to a therapeutic dose of ultraviolet A light. This treatment, called *PUVA*, is used to treat some stubborn skin conditions such as psoriasis. Patients undergoing this treatment must be very careful to avoid any additional exposure to ultraviolet radiation.

PSORIASIS. A chronic, noncontagious skin condition characterized by red scaly patches overlaid with thick, silvery gray scales. It results from unusually rapid turnover of epidermal cells that do not mature properly.

PUVA. *See* PSORALENS.

RADIATION. The process of emitting energy—in the form of X rays, visible light, shortwave radio waves, ultraviolet rays, or any other electromagnetic rays—from one source or center. In medicine, these rays may be used for treatment or for diagnosis.

RADIATION ONCOLOGIST. *See* Radiotherapist.

RADIATION THERAPY. The use of electromagnetic rays (or radiation) in the treatment of disease.

RADIOACTIVE. Emitting radiant energy.

RADIOCURABLE. Curable by radiation alone.

RADIOLOGIST. A physician who specializes in various kinds of body imaging, most of which make use of radioactive substances.

RADIONUCLIDE. An unstable nucleus, together with its orbital or radioactive electrons. Sometimes called *isotope*.

RADIOPAQUE. Opaque to radiation. Any contrast medium that is taken internally to block X rays so that body structures show up clearly on an X-ray film is radiopaque. (Barium is an example of a radiopaque substance.)

RADIORESISTANT. Resistant to the effects of radiotherapy. The term is used to characterized cancers that do not always shrink under radiation.

RADIOSENSITIVE. Sensitive to the effects of radiotherapy. The term is used to characterize a cancer that usually responds well to radiation.

RADIOTHERAPIST. A physician who is specially trained in radiotherapy.

RADIOTHERAPY. *See* RADIATION THERAPY.

RECURRENCE. Return of symptoms or tumor (whether or not expected). A tumor may recur in the site of origin or elsewhere, if it has metastasized.

RED BLOOD CELLS (RBC). Small disk-shaped cells that float in blood and contain hemoglobin. They are responsible for the color of the blood, the transport of oxygen to the tissues, and the removal of carbon dioxide from tissues.

RED BLOOD COUNT (RBC). The number of red blood cells per cubic centimeter of blood.

REGIONAL INVOLVEMENT. Spread of cancer from the primary site to adjacent areas.

REGIONAL PERFUSION. Chemotherapy directed with a catheter to a limited area of the body, in order to destroy cancer tissue with minimal damage to normal tissue.

REGRESSION. Shrinkage of cancer growth.

REMISSION. The disappearance of signs and symptoms of cancer.

RESECT. To cut off or excise a segment of a body part or organ.

RESECTABLE. Amenable to surgical removal.

RETINA. Thin tissue found in the innermost lining of the eyeball. It receives the image that the lens has refracted or bent. The retina is composed of many nerve endings and transmits visual stimuli to the brain.

RETIN-A.® *See* TRETINOIN.

RETINOL. A form of vitamin A found in many cosmetics. It has never been demonstrated to work in the same way as tretinoin.

RISK FACTOR. Something that increases a person's chances of getting a particular illness or condition.

RT. Radiation therapy.

Rx. Treatment.

SCAN. A computerized picture of an organ or part of the body, such as the bones, liver, or brain. Radioactive substances are sometimes injected into the patient prior to the scan; these concentrate in the sections of the body to be scanned, thereby improving the image produced.

SCLERA. White of the eye.

SEASONAL AFFECTIVE DISORDER (SAD). Disturbance of mood and behavior that (in the Northern Hemisphere) only occurs in the fall and winter. Therapy involves the use of full-spectrum bright artificial light.

SEBUM. An oily substance produced by the skin.

SENILE KERATOSES. *See* ACTINIC KERATOSIS.

SIDE EFFECTS. Temporary results of drugs or radiation other than the expected curative effects. These problems occur when a treatment affects healthy cells in the body. Common side effects from chemotherapy for cancer are fatigue, nausea, vomiting, decreased blood cell counts, and mouth sores.

SILICONE. Synthetic plastic that can be injected into wrinkles or deeper furrows to smooth them out. It has not received FDA approval for this purpose.

SKIN GRAFT. Skin that is moved from one part of the body to another.

SNOW BLINDNESS. *See* KERATOCONJUNCTIVITIS.

SOLAR KERATOSES. *See* ACTINIC KERATOSIS.

SOLAR LENTIGINES. Brown, flat spots on the backs of the hands and on the face that look like large freckles. They are the result of UVR exposure. Sometimes called *liver spots*.

SONOGRAM. A computer picture that uses ultrasound (high-frequency sound waves) to examine the position, form, and function of anatomical structures. The ultrasound vibrations (or waves) are sent through various parts of the body to create a picture of various layers of the body's interior. A sonogram is the record of these ultrasound tests.

SPF (SUN PROTECTION FACTOR). Ratio of the amount of energy required to produce a minimal sunburn through a sunscreen product to the amount of energy required to produce the same minimal sunburn when no sunscreen protection is present. The Skin Cancer Foundation recommends that everyone use a sunscreen with an SPF of 15 or more, and that it be applied often.

SQUAMOUS CELL CARCINOMA (SCC). A type of skin cancer that begins in the squamous cells of the epidermis.

SQUAMOUS CELLS. Flat cells that make up most of the epidermis. They are situated above the basal cell layer.

STABILIZATION. The state in which a disease or tumor remains the same, without shrinking, growing, or spreading.

STAGE. The extent of the disease.

STAGING. Careful evaluation to determine the extent of a patient's disease.

STRATUM CORNEUM. The top layer of skin. Sometimes referred to as the *horny layer*.

SUBCUTIS. The layer of skin under the dermis. Sometimes referred to as *subcutaneous fatty tissue*.

SUNBURN. A pink color, or scarlet hue along with a warm, tingling discomfort, often accompanied by mild swelling. Depending on skin type and amount of exposure, sunburn can be painful and serious.

SUNSCREEN. A specially formulated substance that, when applied to the skin, either absorbs or reflects the sun's rays, blocking the rays from penetrating the layers of the skin. Chemical screens are generally colorless or a light white color and contain ingredients that filter and absorb the energy from the sun. Physical screens are usually opaque and contain ingredients that reflect and scatter solar rays away from the skin.

SUNSTROKE. *See* HEATSTROKE.

SUNTAN. The result of ultraviolet radiation stimulation of melano-cytes, which then produces melanin, darkening the skin.

SURGERY. Practice of treating diseases, injuries, or deformities by operating, using manipulation or instruments.

SUTURES. Surgical stitches used to bring together two surfaces.

SYMPTOM. A sign or indicator of a disease or change in condition, as perceived by the patient and/or others.

SYSTEMIC. Of or pertaining to the whole body rather than to one part of it.

SYSTEMIC DISEASE. A disease that affects the whole body rather than just one portion of it.

SYSTEMIC LUPUS ERYTHEMETUS (SLE). A chronic inflammatory disease that can affect many systems of the body. Many people who have SLE are extremely sensitive to sunlight and to any other form of ultraviolet radiation; exposure can cause symptoms ranging from a minor flare-up to a serious exacerbation of the disease.

TANNING DEVICE. An artificial source of ultraviolet radiation (usually confined to emitting UV-A), which many people use to get suntans. Dermatologists and the FDA warn that these devices are not safe.

T CELLS. Stimulated by antigens to circulate throughout the body, they are important to the immune system.

TELANGIECTASIA. Fishnetlike display of "broken" blood vessels, often the result of exposure to ultraviolet radiation.

TISSUE. A collection of cells similar in structure and function.

TOMOGRAPHY. A diagnostic technique that combines computers and

X-rays to obtain a highly detailed image of the section of the body being studied. Tomograms usually make use of contrast dye.

TOPICAL. Applied to the surface of the body.

TOPICAL CHEMOTHERAPY. Treatment of skin cancer by application to the skin or body surface of anticancer drugs in a lotion or cream formula.

TOXIC. Poisonous.

TOXIC REACTION. A serious side effect or reaction that may be quite dangerous.

TRETINOIN. A vitamin A derivative that is synthesized chemically and has been used for a number of years to treat acne. Available only by prescription, it has demonstrated success in treating sun-damaged skin for symptoms of photoaging.

TUMOR. Swelling or enlargement due to abnormal overgrowth of tissue. *Neoplasm* refers to tumors that are composed of new and actively growing tissue; their growth is faster than that of normal tissue and serves no useful purpose. Tumors can be either benign or malignant. Cancer cells often form a mass or tumor.

TILS: (TUMOR-INFILTRATING LYMPHOCYTES). White blood cells that are part of the immune system and that can be extracted from a cancer patient's tumor and then grown in interleukin to boost their potency. They are then injected back into the patient.

ULTRASOUND. *See* SONOGRAM.

ULTRAVIOLET RADIATION (UVR, UV-A, UV-B). Solar or artificial radiation of a certain range of wave frequencies. Ultraviolet radiation represents 6 percent of the total solar energy reaching the earth's surface. Three types of UVR are emitted from the sun: UV-A, UV-B, and UV-C. Most of the UV-C never penetrates the atmosphere. UV-B, which represents 0.5 percent of the total solar energy reaching earth, can penetrate the top two regions of the skin and cause redness and burning. UV-A represents 5.5 percent of the total solar energy reaching earth; it is of much lower intensity but can penetrate the third region of the skin, the dermis.

VEIN. A blood vessel that carries blood from tissues to the heart and lungs.

VITAMIN D. A naturally occurring substance that the body uses to achieve the absorption of calcium from the intestinal tract and to ensure the healthy development and growth of bones. Sunlight manufactures vitamin D in the skin, where it is then absorbed into the body. Many foods today are fortified with vitamin D, and supplements are also available.

VITAMINS. Compounds that, in small quantities, are essential for the normal growth, maintenance, and functioning of the body. Vitamins are obtained from well-balanced diets, but many healthy people need vitamin supplements.

VITILIGO. A skin disease characterized by irregular patches of various sizes that are totally lacking in pigment, often with dark borders. The unpigmented patches are extremely sensitive to UVR.

WHITE BLOOD CELLS (WBC). Several blood-cell types that contain no hemoglobin and are active in response to disease, injury, and medication. White blood cells are about one-third larger than red blood cells, and they act against infection.

WHITE BLOOD COUNT (WBC). The number of white blood cells per cubic centimeter of blood.

WORK-UP. The combined results of a medical examination and tests (some of which may be done in a hospital), used to arrive at a diagnosis and a complete medical picture of the patient. *See also* STAGING.

X-RAY. A type of radiation that can be generated by a machine to help make diagnoses and to treat cancer. It enables physicians to visualize the interior portion of a person.

Index